DEADLY NEGLECT

APATHY & DENIAL VS. ACT OF GOD

by Dr. Jim Blair

NOTICE

ALL RIGHTS RESERVED. This book contains material protectd under International and Federal Copyright Laws and Treaties. Any unauthorized reprint or use of this material is prohibited.

No part of this book may be reproduced or transmitted in any form or by any means electronic or mechanical, which also includes photocopying, recording, or by any information storage and retrieval system without express written permission from the author/publishers.

DISCLAIMER

The information presented within this book represnets solely the view of the author and publishers and is intended for informational purposes only as of the date of publication. The author is active in a number of healthcare domains, and this book does not represent the view of the author's organizational associations. The use of "we" is a substitute for "I" in all cases.

This book offers no private or professional advice. The reader is encouraged to use good judgment when applying information herein contained and to seek advice from a qualified profesional, if needed. The author and the publishers shall in no event be held liable for any loss or other damages, including but not limited to special, incidental, consequential, or other damages. The reader is responsible for any subjective decision made as to the content and/or its use.

For questions or comments regarding any aspects of this book, Dr. Blair welcomes you to contact him at james.blair@chcer.org.

©2011 Dr. Jim Blair. All Rights Reserved.

Dedication

This book is dedicated to a group of courageous nurses who: First, braved the horror of treating frail vulnerable patients, all trapped in disintegrating hospital facilities savaged by destructive winds and inundated by flood waters; Second, volunteered courageously for an investigation which would place them in a position of having to recount those horrible experiences; and Third, for volunteering to participate in such an investigation in a hostile atmosphere characterized by accusations of murder and neglect by caregiver colleagues. To Marti Jordan PhD who agonized over the prospect of putting these nurses through what must be the emotional trauma of re-living those terrifying experiences. Dr. Jordan was not among those who experienced these events first hand but was to become a victim of Katrina through her investigative work. She now finds it unacceptably painful to engage in the retelling of her story. The author will do his best to convey the spirit and driving force which motivated this courageous band of Nurses to participate — *"so this would never happen again."*

Contents

Introduction 1
1. Setting the Stage 3
2. All-Hazards Readiness is a Dynamic Process 9
3. Not Your Everyday Dissertation 13
4. Findings 17
5. Discussion 61
6. Could This Happen Again? 65
7. The "Weakest Link in the Homeland Security Chain".. 69
8. Where is the *Adult* Supervision? 77
9. Reap the Wind 85
10. Lessons Not Learned! 91
11. The All-Hazards Perfect Storm 103
12. Final Note 109
Appendices 113
References 125
Author Profile 152

Introduction

The Center for Health Care Emergency Readiness (CHCER) in Nashville, Tennessee, was established as a partnership of concerned healthcare professionals. Our common experience in hospital and healthcare administration convinced us that huge gaps existed in the Homeland Security readiness posture in the nation's healthcare industry.

This focus brought our attention to a contemporaneous interest of nursing in the Homeland Security domain. News of the establishment of Masters and PhD degrees in nursing with a concentration in Homeland Security (first in the nation) at the University of Tennessee at Knoxville (UTK) led us to consider a joint conference opportunity. A subsequent visit to the UTK College of Nursing provided a comprehensive understanding of the program and an ensuing meeting with PhD candidate Marti

Jordan and the collection of additional in-depth information on her project.

Chapter One
Setting the Stage

The greater New Orleans area has a long history of violent storms. Between 1852 and 2006 there have been twelve major hurricanes (category 3 or greater) passing within 100 miles of the city. The area is also subject to other natural flooding events associated with Mississippi river floods. Manmade attempts to reduce the consequences of one or the other threats have been mixed.

Recent efforts to prepare for and respond to these threats have attracted costly regional planning projects focused on vulnerability mitigation and robust response actions. The Disaster Mitigation Act (DMA) of 2000 tasked states to reduce vulnerabilities associated with the area's known threats.

The Federal Emergency Management Agency (FEMA) funded the 2004, Southeast Louisiana Catastrophic Hurricane Plan (PAM). The plan's exercise scenario incorporated evidenced-based experiences with assumptions about slow-moving category 3 hurricanes and the probable impact on New Orleans. Exercise PAM was only the most recent effort to test what experts projected as the consequences of a storm of this magnitude. Virtually every known problem in dealing with a large hurricane surfaced in spades; evacuation, law and order, sheltering, search and rescue and the ever present need for effective leadership.

The PAM Exercise was concluded more than a year before Katrina made landfall. Months following the exercise were devoted to "fine tuning" action plans developed during the exercise. Healthcare organizations held conferences and shared information which focused on the Exercise findings and stressed the need to implement appropriate action.

Ironically, the picture which developed out of the PAM exercise was to be a "near clone" of what actually became hurricane Katrina. The city had experienced serious flooding in the past. Lessons learned from the 2001 Tropical Storm Allison with its extensive flooding and damage to the hospital and healthcare system in Texas was fair warning to authorities.

It is difficult to measure PAM's immediate impact on

preparedness, however there was a sense that something was being done to make the area safer for its citizens.

The Nation needed to prepare for and respond to growing numbers of threats: the first Twin Towers bombing; the Oklahoma City Federal Murrah Building bombing; the 9/11 terrorist attacks; occasional domestic violence and experience with more robust natural disasters led to the establishment of the Department of Homeland Security (DHS).

The establishment of the DHS was an enormous undertaking which led to the restructuring of the Administrative Branch of the government not seen since the establishment of the Department of Defense (DoD) more than five decades before.

The birth of the new Department was/is characterized by a long and painful gestation period resulting in a number of congenital malformations. The merger of Public Health and Healthcare has been troublesome. A weak and underfunded Department of Homeland Security Health Affairs and a fumbled hand-off of major roles and responsibilities to the Department of Health and Human Services (DHHS) have retarded the pace of expected implementation.

A fragmented Congressional oversight structure has

added to the sector's difficulties. The Public Health and Healthcare Sector does not have a corner on this aspect of oversight, it is pervasive.

The DHS has the broad mission to protect the nation from both manmade and naturally occurring events. Stated strategic goals include: awareness, prevention, protection, response, and recovery. Preparedness for and response to hazardous events is considered a "Local Responsibility," with assistance provided from other levels of government if needed. While the DHS has delegated substantial elements of the operational and oversight mission for the Public Health and Healthcare Sector to the Department of Health and Human Services (DHHS), it retains significant authority and responsibility for the sector's mission accomplishment.

To do their part, hospitals and healthcare organizations are expected to maintain their decades old mission to prepare for natural disasters and other mass casualty producing events.

More than a decade earlier President Reagan's Executive Order 12656, November, 1988 called for a plan to meet the looming threats from "post-cold war" Weapons of Mass Destruction (WMD) falling into the hands of non-state terrorists. The Department of Health and Human Services (DHHS) was tasked with the development of a comprehensive plan to mobilize the Nation's healthcare industry to meet the immediate challenges posed by emerging terrorist threats.

By 2005 the national strategy for Homeland Security protection had matured through a number of levels from the Federal Response Plan (FRP) to National Response Plan (NRP). Pivotal to the success of the response plans at all levels is the adoption of the Nation Incident Management System (NIMS)

The overarching theme imbedded in the NRP and NIMS is a concept of a good-faith partnership between and among the nation's economic sectors. Hospitals demonstrated their readiness through an Accreditation process (External Evaluation Mechanism) contracted by the Center for Medicare and Medicaid Services (CMS), an arm of DHHS.

In late summer of 2005 *all hospitals in New Orleans* had, through the Accreditation process, been deemed in compliance, ready to meet their roles and responsibilities in the event of an "all-hazards event."

Hurricane Katrina was tracked by authorities for days prior to landfall and information on the storm's speed, strength, and every movement was available to all in real time.

The overall chaotic response to the storm's landfall and subsequent flooding is extensively documented. Our focus is on the Public Health and Healthcare sector. Was there a false sense of security promoted by so many objective signs that the healthcare community was prepared? Was there a false assumption that Exercise PAM had measurably improved the region's readiness to deal with this area's most threatening natural disaster scenario?

Chapter Two

All-Hazards Readiness is a Dynamic Process

All-Hazards Readiness is not a destination, it is a journey. Those entrusted with oversight for the safety and security of the nation's most vulnerable populations, sick and injured inpatients have a heavy burden. Hospitalized individuals in today's facilities have increased acuity (sickness), and are often dependent on sophisticated equipment to keep them alive.

The federal agency responsible for insuring the quality, safety and security of the nation's patient populations is the Department of Health and Human Services (DHHS). This Agency relies on contractual arrangements at state, federal or private sector levels for "hands-on" evaluation of such care.

One important aspect of this evaluation centers on the provision of a safe and secure locus of care. The overarching theme embedded in the standards used to evaluate disaster preparedness and response is a timely, informed decision by hospital authorities to either "protect in place or evacuate."

To protect in place means just that. The decision-making matrix for that judgment has evolved over the years to adjust for significant changes in healthcare environments.

Gone are the days when patients would linger for weeks in a hospital bed. Today's hospital census is considerably different, characterized by the phrase "sicker and quicker." This increased acuity (sickness) level of patients has an important impact on bed availability needed for crisis events "surge capacity." The number of patients who may be comfortably discharged is limited. The remaining numbers of patients generally need some level of life support or are equipment-dependent; respirators, monitoring devices, etc. Decisions associated with patient safety need to be made well before the threat arrives on their doorstep.

Gone are the days when each hospital had its own system of on campus resupply of expended medications, medical supplies and equipment. Labor intensive and expensive supply depots have been replaced by the economic alternative, "just in time deliveries." The financial/

operational impact of the "just in time" mode of resupply it not without its own perils; it has added additional complexity to many crisis response decisions. Paramount among these is the "protect in place" option.

Gone are the days when most healthcare delivery functions were organic (owned by) to the organization. The evolving practice of "outsourcing" functions has reduced the organization's control of the resources needed in times of crisis. The outsourcing organization's commitment to immediate response to a hospital's needs during a crisis has been marginalized by over-subscription of those resources within the larger system. For example: The food service surge commitment may have been made with other facilities and local school buses these plans to use in a crisis may also be committed to others.

Gone are the days when the majority of major decisions, with significant economic impact, are in the direct control of "on the ground" hospital authorities. The evolution away from local control for community hospitals to the control of larger corporate entities has steadily increased over the last decade.

The decision to "evacuate" is no less complex. The availability of dependable transportation, safe and secure routes of evacuation, pre-designated alternative treatment sites capable of meeting the needs of evacuated patients and other stakeholders are but a few of the questions to be answered. Timely informed answers to these questions are not readily available in the middle of a crisis. Comprehensive prior planning is **Essential**. ("You can't change a tire on a moving vehicle").

The stage is set.

Chapter Three
Not Your Everyday Dissertation

Selection of a topic for a doctoral dissertation is one of the most difficult tasks facing a PhD candidate. Selection of a topic in pursuit of a new professional domain is perplexing. Marti Jordan was treading in an area with limited research literature available and fraught with other exceptional challenges. Proper articulation of the initial "purpose statement" goes a long way in developing other elements of a proposed academic investigation.

The stated purpose of the investigation was "to describe the experiences of nurses providing care for patients in hospital facilities in Mississippi and Louisiana during and after Hurricane Katrina." The Research Question: "What was the experience of providing care to patients during and immediately after Hurricane Katrina (between August 28, 2005 and September 12, 2005)?"

The investigation was delimited to English speaking

licensed registered nurses who were over the age of 21. Participants came from a limited subset of nurses who were employed in the facilities prior to the hurricane.

The structure of the research approach was complex. The usual task of finding volunteers to participate in the investigation was complicated by the hostile atmosphere created by the arrest of three hospital-based professional caregivers charged with the murder of their patients during and after Hurricane Katrina.

Finding a group of professional Registered Nurse (RN) caregivers who were willing to participate in an investigation into their hour-by-hour experiences during the crisis was a difficult task. Providing a process which shielded them from future retribution was critical to any successful recruitment. Once these barriers were overcome, finding volunteers who were willing to share those agonizing experiences further complicated the effort.

Research which involves human subjects is guided by a very precise set of protocols to insure the emotional and physical safety of both the human subjects and the researcher.

This research required a structure which would protect all from the physical and psychological risks which fall into number of categories: 1) emotional distress, 2) perceived or real threat to licensee and professional livelihood, and 3) perceived or real threat of incarceration.

The extraordinary care taken in the design of the interview process may be found in Appendices A, B, C, & D.

Mutual trust and common cause go a long way to cement a bond among all involved for such an undertaking.

The next chapter is Doctor Jordan's account of her interviews with the participants. The author has organized the materials into segment but has retained the original text found in the study.

Chapter Four
Findings

INTRODUCTION

This chapter presents the findings of the interpretive analysis with exemplar quotes from nurses about what the experience of providing care during and after Hurricane Katrina was like. Participants will be described by means of demographic characteristics and vignettes. The contextual ground of the experience will also be described and a thematic structure will be presented.

The participants included nine registered nurses: Two nurses had diplomas in nursing, three had Associates Degrees in Nursing, two had Bachelors Degrees in Nursing and two had Masters Degrees in Nursing. Eight were female and one was male. Their ages ranged from 29-61 years. They had been nurses from 5-29 years. All were working in hospitals that lost power, potable water, food and supplies. Five were in facilities that experienced flooding into the building.

PARTICIPANT VIGNETTES

Karen

Karen was interviewed in a FEMA trailer located in a neighborhood in a city in a Gulf Coast state. To get to her interview I drove through neighborhoods that were still gutted seventeen months after Hurricane Katrina. Many of the houses still had orange X's on them where they had been searched for bodies after the floods. The smell of mold was pervasive in the air. Karen told me she was in the hospital from Sunday before the hurricane to the Friday afterwards. Karen chose to work PRN (as needed) when she went back to work after Katrina so she would not be required to go in to the hospital during another hurricane. During the interview, she began crying. After the interview Karen told me that this was the first time she had cried since the ordeal. Karen was very focused on the inability to provide patient care in the usual way without technology and with the issues surrounding patient deaths during the hurricane.

Tamara

To interview Tamara, I drove over 750 miles round trip to where she had relocated after the hurricane. The interview took place in an open office at a private university in an affluent area of a major metropolitan city in the southeastern United States. Tamara told me she moved to a different state so she wouldn't have to work during another hurricane. During the interview she talked a lot about guns, people outside with guns, wishing she had brought her gun to work with her, and those who had brought their guns with them to work. Issues surrounding patient deaths also stood out for her. Tamara was angry and confused that she was told not to care for patients that had been transferred to her hospital because they didn't come with supplies and caregivers.

Rose

Rose was interviewed at a public library. I was stunned to see so many houses along the interstate that were still uninhabited 19 months after the hurricane. Rose left the area for a month after the hurricane and thought about not going back, but she decided that since her kids' school reopened, she would return. Rose went back to the same hospital to work, but it is now owned by a different corporation. Rose talked a lot about patient deaths and how difficult it was to have people in the hospital who were discharged during the hurricane and therefore were considered boarders so they received no nursing care, food, water, or medicine. She just couldn't quite understand how that was reasonable.

Chris

Chris was also interviewed at a public library. Her family was with her at the hospital during and after the hurricane. She was very close to her co-workers and had a very strong faith in God. Unlike the other participants interviewed to this point, Chris did not talk as negatively about the hurricane. She also did not talk about her current employment status. Chris was very focused on how the environment affected her ability to care for patients, specifically intravenous (IV) skills and assessments of the patients.

David

A public library was also the site for David's interview. David talked a lot about the difficulties caring for patients by flashlights or in the dark and the increased responsibilities he had during the storm. These responsibilities included controlling civil unrest and evacuating people to the roof. He also described helicopters flying around the city after the hurricane. He saved a picture he took with his cell phone of a helicopter landing on the roof of the hospital he was working in during the hurricane. He went to work after the hurricane at a hospital that suffered the least and was geographically removed from the part of the city that flooded.

Kathy

Kathy was interviewed at a coffee shop. Her speech was tense during the interview, and she cried several times. Kathy described how difficult it was to care for patients because of the lack of medications, emergency equipment, and supplies. Kathy also talked a lot about evacuating patients and about her ordeals at the shelter to which the patients were eventually evacuated. Kathy went to work at a different hospital a week after the hurricane but is now teaching at a nursing school.

Tonya

Tonya was interviewed at her home in a rural area in a Southern state. She shared that she had previously been interviewed by the local television station and, for privacy reasons, preferred to do the interview in her home. Tonya described her inability to care for patients in the way she had been trained and to prevent patients from dying as agonizing. She also talked about how not being able to provide care to her patients made her feel that she had failed as a nurse. She is now working in a medium sized hospital in a different state. She completed the disaster nursing training offered by the Red Cross after Hurricane Katrina and plans to help in future disasters.

Alice

Alice was interviewed in a conference room of a public building in a city in a Southern Gulf Coast state. Alice talked about how difficult it was for her to not be able to meet her patient's physical needs because of the lack of supplies and the loss of technology. She described the change of mindset related to caring for patients during the ordeal. She is now working as nurse practitioner in a clinic.

Erica

Erica was interviewed at a coffee shop. Erica did not work for a while after the hurricane. She left medical-surgical nursing and went to work as a psychiatric nurse. Erica described in detail what the wind was like when it blew so strong that all the windows on one side of the building exploded. She also talked about how scared she was when evacuees started rioting.

CONTEXTUAL GROUND OF THE EXPERIENCE

The contextual ground of the experience was that of wanting passionately to provide comfort and care to patients during and after Hurricane Katrina. The extreme conditions under which the nurses had to work hindered their efforts at every turn. The hospital environment was perceived as terrifying, chaotic, dangerous, threatening, isolating, and primitive. The environment was such an overwhelming obstacle to care that it was described in every narrative. The environment was related to everything experienced, and the term "Hell" was used to describe the circumstances. Regardless of the stories the participants told, the same themes were reflected.

Extreme Conditions

"Hell" as described by the participants was a place where conditions were so brutal that people were unable to escape from it. After the hurricane made landfall, nurses in hospitals along the Gulf Coast lost resources including water, power, telephones, food, and medical supplies and technology needed to provide care to patients. Heat and humidity was unbearable. Conditions were so restricted that nurses were unable to meet their patients' needs or their own. Lack of sleep led to exhaustion that placed a heavy toll on them physically and emotionally. Alice described it best, "The conditions were deplorable...you've got hunger, heat, fear, anger...none of the toilets work... going into those bathrooms...I thought I was going to throw up...we were in hell."

The nurses were so heavily assaulted by stimuli from the environment that the experiences were often described in vivid detail from a sensory point of view. They described what they saw, what they smelled, what they heard, and what they touched in such detail that I could picture it in my mind during the interviews.

What they saw: "I can still see their eyes."
Nurses talked about visual images of fires burning throughout the city, people standing outside the buildings with guns, people looting buildings, floodwaters seven to fourteen feet high, pieces of buildings flying in the wind during the storm, windows blowing in, and helicopters flying over the city. Karen described what she saw when she went in to assess her patients by flashlight. "Just the looks

on their faces, and, their eyes...I saw their eyes...seeing their...their fear and their...and they're all diaphoretic and those...and their eyes...and I can still see their eyes."

Kathy talked about a fire in the shopping center two blocks from the hospital. "You could look and see that there was something on fire...that night when we were up on the roof it was beautiful...and the fire was gorgeous...it lit the sky up a little bit."

What they smelled: "The rush of odors from the morgue."
Nurses talked about how pungent the smells were inside the buildings as well as outside. Some of the things they remember smelling were fires, decomposing bodies, toxic chemicals, human waste, and sweaty bodies.

Karen described the smells from the morgue when they had to take bodies to it.

It was OR #6 where we had to bring all our expired patients...that caused a lot of anxiety for a lot of us... but the odor and the stench of the morgue...and every time we had to open that door...and that...the...the rush of odor that would come through the hallway... and knowing what that odor was. (Karen)

David talked about the smells inside the building and

outside the building.

> The water that... that flooded around the hospital was filled with every filth and chemical known to man. It was the stinkiest water I've ever smelled in my life. I mean all the sewers were all backed up... none of the toilets worked, so if you had a toilet, it was usually filled with either urine or feces... and you could just smell the smell. (David)

What they heard: "All we heard was helicopters flying and gunfire at night."
Nurses talked a lot about hearing gunshots at various times during the day and night, screams, crying, helicopters, car alarms going off after they flooded, and visitors plotting to get the nurses. Some described what it sounded like when there was complete silence. Gunfire meant different things to different people. To some it was scary and made them wish for a gun for protection. For others it made them angry, because it meant that rescues from the facility would have to stop. Others felt safer knowing there were people in the facility with guns to protect them.

Karen described the sounds she and the other nurses heard after the floodwaters came down the streets and the water started rising. "When the water started to rise,

FINDINGS

everybody's car alarm...every employee...and it was everybody's alarm started going off at the same time...and as the water rose, and then all the car alarms...just having the muffled underwater...and then just silence." Rose talked about the sounds she heard while working the night shift. "It was a little scary...all we heard was helicopters flying, and gunfire at night...and then having people tell us not to got outside because somebody would shoot us standing out there."

What they touched: "It was so warm in the rooms their skin was moist."
Nurses talked about how the environment affected the sense of touch (feeling). The environment was wet and hot. These two descriptions as well as descriptions of humidity came up in the nine interviews over a hundred times.

Tamara described what it felt like in the operating room that had been converted into the morgue, "It was so hot and humid that it was actually raining...and the...the...the shrouds are that plastic stuff...and fortunately we had put some identification inside, because what was on the outside...the written tag...it was ruined. It got...the writing just ran right off. " Chris talked about how moist patients' skin was due to the heat, "It was so warm in the rooms that their skin was moist …and patients were sweating so the IVs would come out…they were sliding out…and because the adhesive tape would not adhere to the skin, so the IVs were like sliding out…so we really had to monitor those to be sure they stayed in."

Not only did the nurses describe the sensory aspects of the experience, they also talked about other conditions they faced while living through the hurricane and the aftermath. Nurses were in buildings that suffered structural damage and had design features that even though they were intended to protect, led to more confinement in the aftermath of the storm. Interior building conditions were barely tolerable due to excessive heat, humidity, and unsanitary conditions.

All the participants talked about the heat and humidity. They described how it affected them personally, and how it interfered with other aspects of their jobs. Power outages and loss or failure of generators coupled with heat in the South in August made conditions unbearable. Several of the nurses described the heat and humidity. David said, "During the day, temperatures on the floor would exceed over a hundred degrees and night wasn't much better… there was no breeze…so it was just a stifling, sweltering heat." Karen described it like this, "The humidity was so

FINDINGS

bad the paper was wilted."

Tamara said, "When you watched it [Katrina aftermath] on television, it doesn't begin to convey how really awful it was. You don't have the oppressive heat and humidity." They all talked about the lack of sanitation also. Hospital stockpiling of contaminated waste and garbage; decomposition of bodies; and hallways, stairwells, and bathrooms overflowing with human excrement led to a stench that attracted Nutria rats seeking higher ground and food. Seeing the rats, which are the size of a small dog, was horrifying for one participant. Alice described the smell of fecal material, "The conditions were deplorable...none of the toilets work...I've been a nurse a long time...real strong stomach...I've cleaned people up, never thought anything about it...But going into those bathrooms...I thought I was going to throw up." Kathy described what it looked like, "No control over anything...all the bathrooms were overflowed...we had excrement in the stairwells."

Tonya described the Nutria Rats that came because of the unsanitary conditions.

I'd heard people talk about Nutria Rats, but I'd never actually seen one, 'cause that's not something you're going to see around a hospital...we were actually containing these things in a stairwell...and they're as big as my Pomeranian and they have big buck teeth and they're a huge rat. (Tonya)

Most nurses reported that the hospitals ran out of food and water. Most hospitals had only planned for a two or three day supply of food and water for a minimal census. Some hospitals had an abnormally high census for the time of year. Others that had planned for minimal people had four to seven times that number. What were not accounted for were evacuees other than patients, which included the families of patients and staff. Flooding of the cafeterias also affected the reserve food supplies.

Most of the hospitals began rationing food the first day and some ran out by Wednesday. David talked about the amount of food and water that was available.

For supper we had half of a sandwich and a...and a piece of fruit...I had to explain to the nurses that we only had two gallons of water for twenty-seven patients for the night...we had to do a med pass on patients... the 9 o'clock, when each patient got exactly one-half of a six ounce Styrofoam cup of water. (David)

Erica added to the description. She said, "We got dry cereal and fruit for breakfast...half a ham sandwich for lunch and

FINDINGS

dinner...in five days I had 16.9 ounces of water."

In summary, the environment evoked fear and contributed immensely to the negativity of the experience. Safety and security and basic physiological needs were not met. The buildings were coming apart while the nurses watched. The heat and humidity were oppressive. Conditions were so extreme that they seemed almost too horrible to be true.

THEMATIC STRUCTURE

Six themes emerged from the participants' descriptions of the experience. Most of the nurses discussed all of these themes during their interview. **The themes were 1) Fear, 2) Blurred Boundaries, 3) Ethical Conflicts, 4) Isolation/Connection, 5) Powerlessness/Power, and 6) No Hope/No Hope.** None of the themes were dominant over the others. All the themes influenced each other. The last three themes were experienced opposites on a continuum. The themes were all interdependent and interconnected and described within the context of caring for patients. The thematic structure is diagrammed in Figure 4.1. (*see page 32*)

While practicing within extreme conditions ("hell"), nurses experienced fear, faced ethical conflicts, and saw

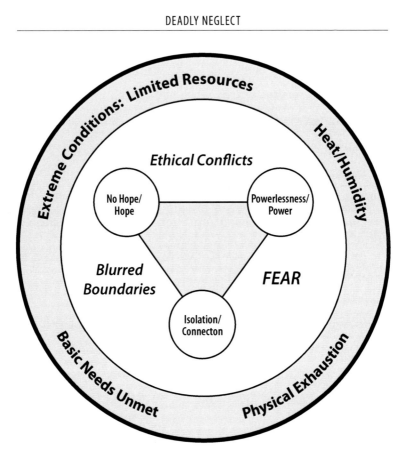

FIGURE 4.1
Thematic Structure: The Experience of Providing Care During and After Hurricane Katrina

the boundaries of nursing blur. During the experience they became physically and interpersonally isolated so they tried to reestablish connection by strengthening bonds with coworkers and with spiritual connections. Continuing and worsening of extreme conditions led to a loss of control and feelings of powerless. To combat this situation and to try and establish power, nurses adapted and improvised to provide the care they felt their patients required. Throughout the experience, hope fluctuated.

Fear: "I really thought we were all going to die."

When describing their experience, participants noted that the environment was threatening. Doors were chained shut from the inside to prevent criminals from breaking in. Predators, such as alligators and stingrays, circled the buildings, and vermin roamed the stairwells unchecked. Interiors without windows were pitch black 24 hours a day leaving nurses with no resources other than hearing or touch once flashlight batteries failed.

Nurses experienced fear of death when they witnessed parts of the buildings that they were in destroyed during the hurricane, and when the levees broke and the flood waters came in. Later they experienced fear when civil unrest elevated, flooding continued, and predators came into the flood waters. Tamara watched the roof peel back and parts of the building being blown out and wondered if they would make it. She said, "I really thought we were all going to die…I didn't think the hospital would be able to maintain through the storm." Alice described the wind blowing out the windows and said, "I had a true feeling that we were going to die."

Just when people thought the storm had passed and they let down their guard, the sense of relief did not last long. Several of the nurses watched the water coming down street after the levees broke and worried the buildings would implode like the Twin Towers on September 11 2001 and feared death. Karen said,

That was the worst part...we saw the water come down the street, and there were white caps coming down the street...and not knowing if it was the beginning of the end...and is this how I was going to die...is this how all of us were going to die...the first thing I thought of was this is how it must have been with 9/11. (Karen)

Most of the nurses reported that they not only felt threats from outside the building but from inside as well. The situation was so unsettling that nurses described it as surreal, like a dream, like watching a movie, and one hoped she would wake up to find the storm gone. Several of the nurses described the pervasiveness of the violence that they witnessed and the lengths they had to go to protect themselves.

They [hospital administrators] had locked all the doors, and there were actually hoodlums...they were just criminal element, outside with guns, trying to get in. It never occurred to me, never in a million years would it have occurred to me to bring my gun to work with me...fortunately, some people did bring their guns. And I mean it was vigilante time. (Tamara)

David added to the description, telling what he heard. *In the city...it felt like...it felt crazy. And what was even worse was hearing the shots...because you would hear people shooting...knowing that people with guns out there were shooting... (David)*

Kathy described how rescue operations were thwarted after someone shot at the helicopter.
We were pulling patients out to the dock, and we had to stop because somebody shot at the helicopter. When they wouldn't stop shooting at the helicopter, and they were rushing the helicopter...and then they had to shut everything down because some idiot decides he's going to shoot the helicopter. (Kathy)

Threat from inside the building included fires, hoarding,

and riots. Kathy talked about a fire that started after a power surge: "We actually had a fire break out in the emergency room, because of electrical...it flashed and then came back on, and something caught it on fire here in ER." (Kathy) Several nurses described incidents of violence occurring in the building. David said, "We had instances where families would steal and hoard. So, it was not uncommon that we had to watch our...anything that we set down... if we set it down and did not keep our...our eyes on it, it would become stolen." Alice talked about the riots outside the intensive care unit (ICU). She said, "They were threatening outside...there was, like some rioting going on...we had to worry about our safety from the people that were in...in the hospital." Erica told about a direct threat she received.

You could hear kind of whispers...and I just could almost feel dissention in the air...and just people started gathering and screaming and...and cussing... I got a flashlight shined in my eye, and a male voice said, "There's a nurse. If she leaves, I'm gonna f****** slit her throat. (Erica)

Threats were not only from people, but from unexpected sources as well. These included animal predators and vermin. Particularly frightening were threats from alligators and sting rays which circled the buildings. Tonya said, "And you could take your flashlight and shine it at night, and see the alligators' eyes everywhere." David talked about other predators he saw in the water, "I seen for myself a three-foot wide stingray swimming at the parking lot at the hospital that I was working."

Blurred Boundaries: "We did everything. We did anything. We did what we had to."

Participants reported that during the hurricane they did everything and anything they had to do to care for their patients. Nurses described situations where credentials were ignored and professional boundaries became blurred. They reported that they wore many different hats and had to make many adaptations to carry out their responsibilities. At times, they reported they felt like policemen, patient transporters, and professional movers. While in the hospital during the hurricane, they reported that boundaries became blurred and team work increased, but at times responsibility also increased. During the ordeal, they had to reach out for help from others. Nurses trained patient's family members, staff's family members,

National Guardsmen, and nurses' aides how to help them care for patients because at times they were not physically able to carry on.

During this time lay people were trained to provide care, and doctors did "non-doctor" work. Anybody who was able and willing was trained to help out because the nurses weren't physically able and didn't have the resources to do it all.

Rose, who didn't have a patient assignment but helped with tasks on a unit, reported that she did anything the nurses asked her do to and it ranged from passing out water to wrapping people after they died. She said, "We did anything…We did everything. We started IVs, cleaned patients, gave them water, took vital signs, gave IV pushes, anything…we admitted people who were brought to the hospital right after the storm and we wrapped people when they passed away." Karen added to the description. She said, "It wasn't a status thing…everybody's credentials went out the window. We just did whatever needed to be done. Everybody worked well as a team."

Not only did the boundaries blur between nurses and lay people, other allied health workers, and doctors, but the responsibilities added to the nursing work load included moving equipment, policing hallways, and transporting patients.

David describe the experience of moving things up when the flooding started.

The water was coming in, so we had to get our critical services up. We had to get, we had to work really fast to get ER, our lab services, our cafeteria...we had to get all that the sixth floor. And so that was, that was the job. To get all that secure...pharmacy had to be moved...(David)

David also talked about the added responsibility that came while trying to maintain control in the chaos.

I had to try to maintain an atmosphere of calm and some authority over the situation...You defused every situation you come to. You just went around...that's all you did was just defuse, defuse, defuse...You policed, like you would children. (David)

He also talked about the role changes he went through.

When the helicopters started coming, my role changed from a nurse to a transporter. I spent from Wednesday... Wednesday morning to Friday morning transporting patients. I did not sleep, because my goal was to get everybody out. (David)

Increased responsibilities not only came with trying to maintain control of the chaos, it came as a result of the situation they faced. Rose described incidents where they experienced increased responsibility. She said, "It's not nursing like I have ever experienced before…you had to make many more decisions on your own, what was good for the patients, and you…you just didn't have the…anybody to fall back on."

Boundaries not only blurred between nurses and the people they enlisted to help as caregivers, the boundaries between being a caregiver and a patient blurred when nurses succumbed to the extreme conditions and became patients themselves. Nurses described how they were exposed to horrific environmental conditions, and were unable to meet their basic physiological needs. Further, they described daily exposure to threats and death, and that their bodies were in a state of starvation and dehydration. Tamara, Kathy, and Tonya described their own personal experiences with becoming patients. Karen and Kathy described incidents where they watched other nurses becoming patients. When the nurses became patients, they were forced into a role change from nurse to patient.

Four of the nurses described the experience of nurses

succumbing to environmental factors and becoming patients. Most of the nurses experienced dehydration, one was floridly psychotic, and one described the experience as being like that malnourished person from third world countries experience.

Several nurses described what it was like when the nurses started becoming sick and their roles changed from nurse to patient. Tonya said, "At first you had so much adrenaline going that you felt like...you can just do anything...but then you started to wear down. And one by one, some of our nurses started getting sick and dehydrated."

Kathy talked about a nurse that had a psychotic break.
One of our nurses that night started going down. We just started IVs on her...We had already lost one nurse as far as she started hallucinating. She had...voices that she was hearing...she was just total psychotic. You could look at it in her face and it was just a whole different person there. (Kathy)

Kathy and Tonya describe their own experience of becoming a patient.
When I got up there, I didn't feel good. Something just didn't feel right. I felt bad...I remember leaning up

against the wall. And the next thing I realized I was out on the balcony, laying on a mat...and a doctor was starting an IV on me. (Kathy)

Tonya told about her physical condition during and after the experience.
I literally quit going to the bathroom. Most of us did...I don't remember anything but waking up and laying on the ground and seeing a propeller over me, right beside the helicopter...I was severely dehydrated. I had lost ten pounds in a week. When I got back home...try to eat a bite of food...throw up. Stomach couldn't take it. Got used to having nothing. (Tonya)

Ethical Conflicts: "What makes one patient more important than another?"

Decisions needed to be made and nurses were often forced to make decision when no good choices were available. Some nurses made choices to rise above the bad decision(s) and do the right thing, as they perceived it, no matter what they were told to do. Other nurses, who had to make bad choices, later made career changes so they would not have to be in a position to make those kinds of decisions again.

Participants described this theme with great emotion. Some were angry at the decisions made for them or for the positions that they were put in, while others did not understand them. I believe most of them had to look at situations they had never faced before or ever thought they would have to face. Kathy talked about a conflict between two nurses during a code.

> *They were going to take this man's oxygen away. And the nurse who was assigned to him said, "But if you take his oxygen away, he's going to die." And it got to be a battle between two nurses, "But if I don't put it on this lady over here in the code, she's going to die." And one nurse finally said, "But what makes that patient more important than this one? How do you decide in this situation who's more important?"* (Kathy)

Tamara described the dilemma of not being able to care for patients who had been transferred into her hospital. She said, "Our CEO, decided that the medicine that we did have in the pharmacy would be for our patients and they were not going to take care of these [transferred] patients. They were just providing shelter."

Tamara and Rose describe instances where

administrators made choices to discharge people when the people had nowhere to go. They could not understand this decision. Tamara said,

> We didn't have enough water...enough food...I got very, very concerned when the CEO said, "We're going to have to just start telling some people they have to leave." ...and some of the doctors came in and started discharging their patients. I said, "Where are you going to send those patients? I mean, so Grandma...now you say she couldn't go home Friday, but she can go home now, and she has no home? (Tamara)

Rose provided additional detail. She said,

> Some people were just boarders...[they were] discharged from the hospital but had no where to go...we weren't allowed to do anything to them...you discharge them but they don't have anywhere to go, so they're not really discharged to me. I mean, how do you give somebody prescriptions and tell them, "Go." Where? There wasn't anywhere to go. So how do you discharge somebody? (Rose)

Tonya talked about wrestling with the dilemma of possibly having to choose between her own life and the lives of her patients. She said, "I remember ambuing patients until I thought to myself, 'I cant' believe this might come down to me or my patient. How can I choose?'"

Isolation/Connection: "We were an island"/ "We just stuck together like glue"

Many of the nurses were in buildings that were surrounded by flood waters. Several described it as feeling like they were on an island. Others described it as feeling like they were stuck, isolated, and cut off from everything. When participants looked outside they were unable to see anything on the ground or any people outside. Not only were they in buildings surrounded by water, they also had no telephone service or cell phone signals. Because of this participants were unable to call out and nobody could call in.

Several of the nurses described isolation in the physical sense as if they were on an island. Karen said "we were under nine feet of water, and we were an island." David said "you could look out over the city, and you would feel that you were in a…in a lake, and all these little islands that were houses were all around you."

Rose, who had claustrophobia in the past, felt stuck

and scared. She described it like this, "we couldn't use the elevators, we couldn't take the stairs. We were basically stuck. It was very scary. I don't think I have ever been that scared. I don't like to be stuck anywhere."

Others felt the isolation as a loss of interpersonal connection. David said,

> Knowing that my family did not know whether I was alive or dead...there was no way I could call them or talk to them. There was no cell signals...No cell phone worked. There was absolutely no communication with our families. (David)

Rose said, "It [loss of power] just cut us off from everything. We were just cut off from information...any kind of way." Participants described connection as sticking with their friends and supporting each other, forming support groups to talk about feelings and the situation they were in, and as strengthening bonds they had with people they had worked with for a long time. During the hurricane, staff at the hospitals worked together, ate together, slept together, cried together, and were scared together.

Alice and Kathy described the connection they had with people. Alice said, "When I got to the break room about 7pm...one of my long long time friends was there...

and, oh my gosh, we just stuck together like glue, said "Okay, let's both do night shift together; we're going through this together." Kathy said, "And one particular physician…we sat there and we talked for hours…and what was important at this point. What was going to happen when we got out of here and the hope that it…it made it a whole lot more bearable. It was just a bonding that I'll never forget."

Rose and Chris were friends. They talked about the support they received from the nurses they worked with in their department who were sent to the floors as extra help for the staff nurses and how it helped them get through the time they were at the hospital after the storm. Rose said, "We stayed…we slept in the area…so we had ourselves to rely on. And we kind of stuck together. There wasn't anytime that we were alone, without our friends." Chris added to the description, "We're such a close knit group, that we relied on each other for sanity. Our friends were there… we were a close group of people. We had our talk sessions, our talk sessions every night when we would come back to our rooms, probably 2…3 o'clock in the morning."

David also talked about the support he received from co-workers who were like a second family to him and how it helped him get through the ordeal.

> *Whenever we wondered if we were going to make it or not you would talk to people around you. Everybody would try to help everybody else. We'd all worked together there for more than...for almost a complete year. So this even pulled us together ...it helped relieve stress. We'd talk to each other about what was going on...bounce ideas off each other and just talk to each other about what had happened. (David)*

Spiritual connections also helped Tonya cope with the situation.

> *What finally gave me peace was I got down on my knees and I prayed to God and told Him I wasn't as strong as I thought I was, and that even as a Christian when you're put in...in that situation...I said, "I can't do this anymore. I just can't."...And I felt like God sent me...sent me the message...I may not have been there to help them medically...but maybe I was to help them spiritually... so then my whole focus change... off of nursing...which I was still doing...but praying with these patients...and talking to family members and visitors...and started singing gospel songs, and everything just kind of changed. (Tonya)*

FINDINGS

Powerlessness/Power: "I felt like a failure in every sense of the word."/"We just had to pave our own road."

Participants described the care they provided to patients as primitive due to the lack of technology, resources, and supplies. Some felt that using only the most basic nursing methods to care for patients was agonizing. To Karen it was distressing to not be able to care for patients in the way she had been trained.

> We basically used up all those supplies. And then it came to a point where we just didn't have any...any more morphine...we didn't have any more Tylenol. We didn't have any more linen. We had no running water...I felt like a failure in every sense of the word... it was an overall sense of failure...and not being able to have anything to just take care of patients...and then you don't have a purpose. (Karen)

Lack of supplies, resources and technology affected how the nurses did their jobs and forced them to go back to skills they described as primitive, basic, and archaic in the dark or with flashlights. Chris said,

> We had to incorporate the skills that we had acquired in nursing school. The situation was complicated

because you had to bring out skills that you had not used, primitive skills...it made you think and use skills which today's technology have kind of taken away from us. (Chris)

David talked about what it was like to work in the dark. *We had to do everything by flashlight...so, for the majority of the night, we had to sit in our stations with the...with our flashlights off, listening for our patients... It was just basic nursing care. It was down to just basic nursing, giving medications, giving out water, and providing as much comfort as you could. (David)*

Nurses reported having to return to "old school" methods and to provide care without technology. Through improvising they were able to provide the care they felt the patients desperately needed, and in the process of doing this, restored feelings of efficacy in themselves. Alice said,

Patient care was pretty much just...it wasn't happening...Our monitors didn't work...you couldn't do anything that you were used to doing...we just had to pave our own road...I went back to...the very basics of nursing care...and to provide comfort...I think I made

comfort like my number one priority for my patients. (Alice)

Tonya described ways they improvised. She said,
We ran out of linens, so as the patients, needed to be changed, or had bowel movements, we ended up using curtains. We cut them down and cut them...sheets off beds that might have been on the other floors that were not occupied. (Tonya)

Karen added more detail about improvisations. She said,
We basically were squeezing bags [of pressors] into patients...we had no suction...our ventilator patients that were in...in CHF and pulmonary edema...we actually used the bulb suction for infants...and would put a Foley catheter on the end...making stretchers out of sheets...we went to the OR and got...we got the, 3000cc, liter bags of saline that we use for bladder irrigation, we used that to...to...to bathe patients, to, rinse them off. (Karen)

Feelings of power were also restored by affirming that you were in control and you were going to take care of yourself. Kathy equated feeling like a drug dealer as having power and this is how she described it:

I've got twenty-five 50mg Demerols stuck it in the top of my scrub [to give patients who needed them], and I walked around for two days with 50mg Demerol in my chest...we just kept count. Because they'd come find me and they'd go, "We need another one."...I felt like a drug dealer. (Kathy)

No Hope/Hope: "Were we going to live or die?"/ "God's not done with me yet."

With dwindling hope and conditions worsening, the participants not only faced threats coming at them from outside the hospital but from inside as well. Lack of resources (food, water, sanitation) prevented them from meeting their own basic physiological needs, and watching their patients die made them lose hope and question whether they would survive.

There was a lot of anxiety not knowing...were we... were we...you know...all perish?... and when patients started to expire because of lack of power and supply and food and everything...we had know idea how long what we had was going to last...And how long everybody could...could make it, including staff. (Karen)

Tonya added to the description. She said,
> You didn't know if you was going to get out alive or not...the situation was getting so desperate. Under conditions like that you were more just...just overwhelmed at times....I knew if we didn't get out of there and get these patient's out pretty soon, we were all going to die. (Tonya)

Participants discussed how hope came and went. In the face of devastation they tried to remain optimistic. Hearing a radio broadcast instilled hope in one, spiritual connections such as talking to God or having a service by the chaplain helped others.

Tamara described how her hope was restored. She said, "My husband got out and he got to our house...our house was fine...our neighbor's house wasn't fine...we had seven trees in our back yard...they all fell...not one of them hit the house. So I figured, okay, God's not done with me yet."

David revealed that the voice of another nurse's husband on the radio was a ray of hope that changed her whole focus.

> We were able to pick up a radio station, and one of our nurses heard her husband on the radio. And he called

her name, and he said "If you can hear us, just know I love you. We're still looking for you." And that was like hope for everybody. (David)

Karen and Kathy talked about the spiritual connections that helped them get through it.

> The one thing that I did remember that really helped a lot was, a group of therapists that were in the hospital... every day would come at lunchtime and sing... On each unit... And that... that I can tell you was very uplifting, and helped... we had our, our chaplain that was there at the hospital with us, and every day we'd have a service... that did alleviate a lot of stress. (Karen)

Kathy added detail. She said,

> I spent those four or five days talking to God, and every once in a while it would be, "Okay, Lord." And my prayers went from... in the hospital I went from, "Lord, protect us all from the storm," and then it was, "Lord, keep my kids safe." At one point my prayer turned to, "Lord just take me now. Let me go and end this now, I can't do this anymore."... But it got better. (Kathy)

ADDITIONAL FINDINGS

Participants reported that sometime during their experience of Hurricane Katrina they reflected. Some realigned their priorities while others decided that they would never be in the situation again. One grieved losses, while another used it as an experience for growth. Perspective Changes occurred because of nurses' experiences of providing care during and after Hurricane Katrina. Karen said,

> You learn what's important. You value relationships a little bit more, and you're not as selfish... I didn't go back to full-time nursing because I had a lot of anxiety as the new hurricane season approached. I took a PRN job, and that alleviated a lot of the obligation because as a PRN you're not obligated to go to the hospital. I have no... no plans or ever desire to do that again... And I... and I won't. (Karen)

Rose said,

> I would have to think long and hard if I would stay again. I don't know that I would stay. When you wouldn't necessarily have to do anything for somebody to die. Actually, you'd have to do nothing. You don't have to kill them, you just do nothing. You just

let them...I mean, they just would...oh my God...I don't think anybody can imagine how hot is hot. And how draining and...it just was an unbelievable...I don't know. It's hard to even explain. (Rose)

Many talked about the structural damage that the facilities encountered during the hurricane. In the storm ravaged environment, architectural design features, such as hurricane shutters and hurricane windows and layout of departments, to ensure out patient and public access were a serous detriment to the safety and comfort of patients and staff. Every structure in the hospital proved to be vulnerable.

Participants told stories about roofs and windows. Karen said, "The roof caved in, which had one of the generators on that roof. And when the roof caved in, we also had all of our glass windows on the North side of the hospital that blew in." Alice said, "Windows were imploding, we were having to block off doors, and, the...the ceilings were just panels and so they were just falling and falling and falling and falling."

Kathy talked about the material that made up the outside of the new building that had just recently been completed: "Our building was made...what we call foam…part of that started getting some water up it and the front part started collapsing."

Hospital design which placed all the essential services on the first floor was fatally flawed and magnified the ultimate loss of resources when flooding occurred.

> Karen talked about ancillary services. She said,
> *Materials management on the first floor…pharmacy on the first floor…generators on the first floor… Ultrasound, lab, x-ray, everything on the first floor… so we basically had no back-up.* (Karen)

David talked about food supplies. He said,
> *Our cafeteria and our…our resources for the food and for food storage all on the ground floor…when the flood waters started coming in, it came in so fast that only minimal food was able to be taken out of storage and moved up…so automatically [food supply], cut in half.* (David)

Features which were intended to protect the hospital during hurricanes led to more confinement and in turn worsened environmental conditions. Tamara described the windows. She said, "It was so incredibly hot in that building, and it's a modern building…the windows don't open."

Kathy added detail about windows. She said,

> When it got so hot...we decided we needed to do something for patients...the heat was getting intolerable and we noticed there were two windows so we decided we'd just go and break the windows open... unfortunately, the new part of the building had the hurricane proof windows...we took fire extinguishers and were, like bouncing them off those windows and they wouldn't break...one nurse had some sort of jigsaw knife and cut a hole through the window...a hole about golf ball sized...it took her a good couple of hours to cut through that. (Kathy)

SUMMARY

The thematic structure of the experience of providing nursing care during and after Hurricane Katrina was described within the context of caring. The environment was described as "Hell." Working during Hurricane Katrina created an environment where the participants experienced fear, ethical conflicts arose, and the boundaries of nursing became blurred. Along with these conditions they also felt isolated, powerless, and hopeless but didn't give

FINDINGS

up because they tried to reestablish connection, power, and hope. Discussion of the findings, along with implications for theory, nursing practice, education, research, and policy are presented in Chapter Five.

Chapter Five
Discussion

Doctor Jordan's Discussion Chapter is a must read for all those who have direct and/or indirect roles and responsibilities in the broad nursing domain. One is immediately struck by the poverty of literature on the subject. She had to reach out to a range of other health professional domains to fill the gaps.

There appears to be a stark contrast between nurses who have been trained to deal with mass casualties as an integral part of their roles and those who have not. Military nurses who find themselves in similar environments do not appear to sustain the same level of psychological trauma and tend to cope more effectively than those who have not been exposed to such training. We find Dr. Jordan's suggestion that such training would be helpful in preparing nurses for all-hazards mass casualty events to be sound.

Early traditional nursing theory and practice centered on providing for a healing environment for their patients. Dr. Jordan discusses the evolving patient care environment and its increasing reliance on technology. The sudden realization that the most devoted caregiver has diminished control over the greater technological aspects of the patient care is often overwhelming. The long held dominate belief that their role in patient care is key to successful patient treatment outcomes is challenged. For example, loss of electrical power suddenly limits their effectiveness.

Dr. Jordan discusses the wholesale lack of preparedness by hospital authorities. All these nurses found themselves trapped in facilities caring for fragile and equipment-dependent patients. They were in a situation not of their own making. They felt that they had been betrayed by the healthcare system. The hostile environment created by the arrest of other caregivers for allegedly murdering their patients, combined with gag orders from hospital authorities, subjected them to enormous stress. One of the most haunting memories centered on hospital authorities ordering them not to use scarce resources on selected populations within the hospital. This was seen as choosing "who is to live and who is to die." Attempts to

DISCUSSION

follow these orders created ethical and moral conflicts as well as increased threats to their own personal safety and survival.

Dr. Jordan's recommendations in the areas of Public Policy and Future Research focused on efforts to protect caregivers from litigation/prosecution when working in disaster conditions. Also the acute need for a robust all-hazards Nursing education and training component in today's nurse education programs enjoyed a strong recommendation.

Almost six years after the tragic death and destruction wrought by Hurricane Katrina and two years since the publication of "Nursing in Hell The Katrina Experience," Dr. Jordan looks with pride on the exceptional courage of these nine nurses and their willingness to participate in her study. Among her questions: has the pain and self-sacrifice associated with this noble effort produced any measurable change in the area all-hazards readiness? And will nurses and other hospital caregivers better protected when they are faced with the next Katrina?

Chapter Six
Could This Happen Again?

This sobering flashback to the death and suffering in Gulf Coast hospitals-before, during and after — "killer Katrina" — gives us pause and sends us back to look for explanations and speculate on the future.

Five years prior to that fateful day that Hurricane Katrina made landfall the U. S. Congress anticipated the need to prepare for the looming triple threats of the following: Evolving infectious diseases, more frequent and robust natural disasters and mounting evidence that non-state terrorists groups armed with weapons of mass destruction (WMD) posed serious threats to the national landmass.

Personal experiences ("boots on the ground") during the last decade have convinced the author that there are huge gaps in the nation's strategy in Healthcare Homeland Security all-Hazards Readiness.

To those brave nurses who participated in the study

I would say "your experiences" have touched many across the nation. However, the apathy and denial you saw prior to Hurricane Katrina is alive and well across the nation. An additional concern is that both natural and man-made threats are significantly greater today than in the late summer of 2005.

The longer one lives the more he realizes that "where you stand on issues is a function of where you sit." The very nature of the vulnerability assessment process draws you to "what is not there and too often draws you away from what is there."

An extremely important source of information on the evolving **State of the Nation's Homeland Security** level of preparedness comes from the *Government Accountability Office (GAO)* and the *Congressional Research Service (CRS)*

Those who wish to study the issues in depth should review the many GAO and CRS reports available on the subject of "the Nation's Strategy for Homeland Security." Of particular interest are those reports released before Katrina.

These reports are prepared for members of Congress as an adjunct to their other sources of information on specific areas of oversight. Earlier reports, following the 1995 bombing of the Oklahoma City federal Murrah building and 2001 terrorist attacks focus on protecting critical infrastructure and neutralizing the effects of the **Weapons of Mass Destruction (WMD)**. Many have criticized the Congress and GAO for their pre-Katrina focus on WMD, **Chemical, Biological Radiological, Nuclear and Explosive (with or without radioactive materials) (CBRNE)**, perhaps at the expense of preparing for naturally occurring threats.

We posit that, prior to *Hurricane Katrina*, "**Mother Nature" had shown her destructive potential to the area many times over.**

Key Federal legislation followed in the wake of Hurricane Katrina. Two comprehensive laws affecting public health and medical preparedness and response, **The Pandemic and All-Hazards Preparedness Act (PAHPA, PL 109-417)** and **The Post-Katrina Emergency Management Reform Act of 2006 (PKA, Title VI of PL 109-295)**. The later Act reorganized and, within it, the Federal Emergency Management Agency (FEMA). *The PKA also codified the position of DHS Chief Medical Officer, with primary responsibility within DHS for medical issues related to natural and man-made disasters and terrorism.*

Confusion over federal leadership and coordination between and among DHS. DHHS and federal agencies are and have been a problem in the implementation of public health and healthcare Homeland Security protection. **(see CRS R40159)**

An additional rich source of information on the Public Health and Healthcare readiness posture are the serial publication of **"Ready or Not" Trust for America's Health**. These reports are extremely detailed (state-by-state), however, they are subject to an over-reliance on self- reporting and the *researched Indicators change each year*. Following each yearly edition there is a flurry of self-serving media reports generally at the State level reporting information favorable to the state which is often taken out of context.

Chapter Seven

The "Weakest Link in the Homeland Security Chain"

The non-federal hospital and healthcare sector with its public/private blend faces the usual set of regulatory requirements. Effective oversight of the industry has always been challenging. In a free pluralistic health delivery system, governance is fragmented.

State and tribal sovereignty and the stark difference / reality between federal health sector's *mandatory* and the non-federal health sector's *voluntary* compliance for all-hazards preparedness continues to leave huge gaps in the nation's ability to meet today's challenges.

Upward to **90%** of the nation's healthcare response capacity is found in the non-federal sector, (voluntary). The remaining healthcare federal sector, **10%**, (mandatory) provides limited capacity for meeting the nation's need for all-hazards response. It takes more than the federal government to meet the **National Response Framework**

(NRF) mission.

The enormous size and disparate functions represented by the Public Health and Healthcare Sector which employs over 13 million individuals in over a half-million establishments helps one understand the challenge of assembling them into a coherent partnership for Homeland Security Protection. Hospitals represent **2%** of healthcare facilities, however, they employ **40%** of the healthcare human resources.

The Public Health and Healthcare Sector has been/and is characterized as the **"weakest link in the Homeland Security chain."** This Sector is one of eighteen national economic sectors identified as Critical Infrastructures and Key Assets under the National Infrastructure Protection Plan (NIPP).

Congressional oversight for healthcare preparedness for all-hazards events is located in a maze of Committees and Sub-Committees on Capitol Hill.

The post Katrina legislative hearings droned on for months and the GAO reports on what went wrong multiplied. One such Congressional briefing, was based on the issue of "Evacuation of Hospitals and Nursing Homes," February 16, 2006, "Disaster Preparedness: Preliminary Observations on the Evacuation of Hospitals and Nursing

Homes Due to Hurricanes." **The GAO-06-443R** was to explore answers to three questions (1) who is responsible for deciding to evacuate hospitals and nursing homes, (2) what issues administrators consider when deciding to evacuate hospitals and nursing homes, (3) what federal response capabilities support the evacuation of hospitals and nursing homes.

The following background information was presented: (1) Hospitals and Nursing Homes are required to have emergency plans in place, (2) The Centers for Medicare and Medicaid Services requires Hospitals and Nursing Homes which receive reimbursement for care of federal beneficiaries must maintain emergency plans, (3) The Joint Commission on Accreditation of Healthcare Organizations requires that Hospitals and Nursing Homes it accredits maintain emergency plans which include a plan for evacuation.

Answers to the first question were less precise. Hospital and Nursing Home administrators *"often"* have the responsibility for deciding whether to evacuate their patients or to shelter in place during a disaster. State and local governments can order evacuation of the population or segments of the population during emergencies, but healthcare facilities *"may be"* exempt from these orders.

Administrators told the investigators that they evacuate only as a last resort and that healthcare facilities' emergency plans are designed primarily to shelter in place.

Answers to the question about issues which Administrators must consider before evacuating their facilities include adequate "resources" to shelter in place and risk associated with such a move. To consider evacuation they must make prior arrangement for means for such an action. Loss of communications and vital utilities must be considered.

Answers to the third question were interesting. At the time, Department Homeland Security, Department of Health and Human Service and The Joint Commission on Accreditation of Healthcare Organizations doctrine and guidance was not to expect federal assistance for 72 hours.

If I had been a member of the Senate Committee on Health, Education, Labor, and Pensions attending this February 16, 2006 briefing, six months after Hurricane Katrina and five month before the next Hurricane season I am not sure I would have known where to focus my attention.

One difficulty we have with many GAO reports is that they often create more questions than answers. Do

THE "WEAKEST LINK IN THE HOMELAND SECURITY CHAIN"

Hospital and Nursing Home Administrators have the final say on the decision to "shelter in place or evacuate?" Use of words *"often or may be"* lead to confusion. County Officials in Florida did not equivocate, in their testimony that the healthcare administrators made those decisions. Testimony from New Orleans indicated that the Mayor would not let them evacuate. That being the case, where were the voices of Hospital and Nursing Home Leadership? Metropolitan Hospital Council? Louisiana Hospital Association? State Healthcare Trade Organizations? American Hospital Association? National Healthcare Trade Organizations? Federal Healthcare Oversight Agencies? And Congressional Healthcare Oversight Committee Members?

The testimony that *"protect-in-place"* was the dominant assumption which hospital authorities are expected to follow and that *"evacuation is rare,"* also needs explanation. If that were the case, all hospitals must be ready to meet all that is required, all the time, to "protect in place."

One thing we do know is that hundreds of hospital-based caregivers *were placed in life and limb-threatening situations not of their own making.* Their hospital employers were not prepared to *"protect-in-place"* nor prepared to exercise the alternative, *"evacuation."* There was full access to the day-to-day progress of Hurricane Katrina. The question about the accuracy of the warnings was subject to Congressional hearings. The House Select Bipartisan Committee Chairman, Tom Davis, said it all, *"It remains difficult to understand how government could respond so ineffectively to a disaster that was predicted for years, and for which specific dire warnings had been issued for days. If this is what happens when we have advance warning, I shudder to imagine the consequences when we do not."*

We have little doubt that the physical and psychological suffering experienced by our nine nurses may be generalized to the host of caregivers trapped in hospitals across the city and gulf area. As tragic as these experiences were, none faced the additional horror of arrest for killing their frail, helpless charges. This does not mean that their lives have not been changed forever.

We will never know the lasting impact which the *"Katrina Effect"* will have on the nursing profession in the region. We do know that among the nine nurses in the study none will be comfortable in their future in-patient nursing role. A TIME article published one year after Katrina (Tuesday, August 1, 2006) posed the following question and statement, **"Is New Orleans Having a Mental Health Breakdown?" talks of what locals** call "Katrina Brain." **One state mental health expert quoted in a recent local magazine stated "There's no 'post' to the post-traumatic stress syndrome, the stress never goes away."** We do know that as late as last year the city was suffering from a lack of healthcare resources. High on the list of needed care was in the mental health care support area.

The attention given to the arrest of two nurses and a physician for alleged murder of their helpless patients held the attention of the local media and citizens for months following the disaster. Issues associated with *how they found themselves in such a compromised position took a back seat.* Hospital and Healthcare organizations pushed to distance themselves from these caregivers and any culpability associated with placing them in an environment where they were subjected to the specter of such horrible life-death decisions.

Indeed, the industry went on an advertising blitz extolling the personal heroism and organizational effectiveness of their response to the disaster. Little attention was given to the wholesale lack of preparedness and the wisdom of the authorities in their questionable decision to *"protect in place."* Evacuations, in the face of earlier less threatening hurricane were achieved without serious complications including loss of lives and undue physical and emotional trauma to caregivers.

Chapter Eight
Where is the *Adult* Supervision?

The national healthcare media coverage of Katrina had its bizarre moments. In the month after the tragic storm a commentary appeared in one such national magazine **"From advocacy to emergency,"** authored by the president of the Louisiana Hospital Association (LHA) praising the organization's response to Katrina. Nurses trapped in hospitals were not so ready to dismiss the lack of preparedness by the LHA and the Metropolitan Hospital Council of New Orleans. A year later the American College of Healthcare Executives (ACHE) publication, **"Frontiers of Health Services Management"** attempted to explain away the lack of preparedness and endorsed a theme to be better prepared.

The Hospital and Healthcare systems in New Orleans did not need the complex and sophisticated Exercise PAM to alert them to the dangers of flooding along the

Gulf Coast. Tropical Storm Allison's (2001) epic flooding of low lying areas of Houston Texas in general and huge healthcare systems in particular, should have served as an inescapable incubator for serious "lessons learned" for future preparedness.

The Suburban Emergency Management Project (SEMP) Biot Report #216 is among the best coverage of Tropical Storm Allison's devastating impact on Houston's Hospital and Healthcare Systems. The report clearly articulated a series of "lesson's learned," and also included some presence editorial notes: *"External, as well as internal, hospital disasters will become more common as local populations swell in size and built environments constructed in another age (the 1950s and 1960s) experience degrees of failure in the face of natural forces, such as hurricanes and earthquakes. Still, one becomes incredulous to learn that hospitals, known to be sitting in flood plains, would place critical patient-care departments in the basement, as well as electrical switchgear controlling backup diesel gasoline-powered generators two floors above."*

These observations, along with others, should have been a "wake-up call" to others along the Gulf Coast. A year following Tropical Storm Allison (2002) the New Orleans health director questioned the city's hospital executives about their ability to withstand an area flooding event and if their backup generators were at risk under those conditions. He also asked how much it would cost to move them to a protected location. According to a later article (Dr. Sheri Fink) their reply *"They said it would cost millions of dollars and nobody had the money. They thought I was crazy."*

If not elevated to a higher level by New Orleans health authorities, what did external evaluation organizations suggest? Post-Allison all hospitals in the city received an external evaluation and awarded an Accredited/Deemed status with what many identify as a serious gap in sustainability and clear potential danger to all stakeholders.

The Associated Press, October 3, 2005, bold headline, **19 Health Care Facilities Probed in La.** attracted a lot of attention within the hospital and healthcare community. As we will see later this was the start of a long and torturous journey through the legal system.

Twenty years of guidance, Federal all-hazards preparedness and response planning evolved into a comprehensive National preparedness and response plan for known natural and manmade threats *went largely unheeded* by the hospital community.

A year before the 9/11 terrorist attacks, key

representatives of the hospital industry and designated federal agencies met to address the care of mass casualties generated by future manmade or naturally occurring events. There was strong consensus that the group should adopt the Joint Commission Accreditation of Healthcare Organizations' (JCAHO), later TJC, 1998 Environment of Care (EC) Standards and expand involvement with the local community.

The Joint Commission (TJC), until recently, had a monopoly on the provision of External Evaluation of hospitals for eligibility of hospitals to receive reimbursement for care of federal beneficiaries.

Simple enough, theoretically, *Accreditation* is the basis for not only federal reimbursement it also, *"acts as a seal of approval that quality, safe and secure care goes on here."* It is seen as a measure of quality and security and strongly influences insurers and *lending organizations* in their due diligence considerations.

At first glance the external evaluation mechanisms appear to be the *"narrow point in the funnel."* In theory, a TJC survey or other designated survey groups act as a *"trip wire"* for obvious patient and worksite dangers which are the primary responsible of other regulatory entities (Occupational Safety and Health Administration

(*OSHA*), Environmental Protection Agency (*EPA*), Food and Drug Administration (*FDA*), Department of Homeland Security (*DHS*), Nuclear Regulation Commission (*NRC*), etc.). Regulatory enforcement from these entities is fragmented and represents a dazzling array of "some federal, some state and some local regulation authority."

Comprehensive responsibility and accountability for the delivery of patient-centered quality and safety does not exist. **"When everyone is in charge, accountability is an elusive goal."**

A quick review of **GAO-04-850** will give the reader a "point-in-time" reference for the level of oversight performance provided by JCAHO. (One year before Katrina).

Almost three years following Katrina, the summer of 2007, TJC published more explicit guidance to their clients in the form of major revisions to Elements of Performance (EPs) for Standards dealing with Emergency Management.

These EPs strengthened and clarified guidance for hospital *Emergency Management*. Emphasis on the six critical areas of emergency management moved the standards closer to expectations identified in the Center for Medicare and Medicaid Services (CMS) Conditions of Participation

(COPs) and principles embedded in the national strategy for all-hazards protection. The revised Elements of Performance (EPs) are fundamental to and essential for any rational determination of the most difficult of decisions to face hospital authorities/executives in times of crisis, *"Protect-in-place or evacuate."*

One quarter into the 2008 calendar year, these major revised Elements of Performance (EPs) which had been so skillfully articulated as *"predicates to any successful response to future all-hazards crisis" (July,2007)* were not "scored." Client hospitals and healthcare industry trade organizations pressured TJC to drop the requirement for the rest of the year or an undisclosed number of Accredited Facilities would lose their "Deeming and Accreditation status."

None of the extant hospital external evaluation mechanisms (Deeming) for Emergency Management have yet to field an assessment scheme which approximates an acceptable level of readiness envisioned by the National Response Framework (NRF).

The memory of the tragic events of New Orleans' Katrina (2005) faded quickly. Healthcare facilities along the Gulf Coast still have Emergency generators on the lower levels, essential clinical and administrative activities remain subject to nature's wrath. Hurricanes Gustav and Ike devastated hospitals and healthcare facilities and took their toll of human lives, pain and suffering.

Chapter Nine
Reap the Wind

Fast forward to 2010: If we could assemble that brave group of nine Nurses and give them an update on events following their "Katrina Experience" and discuss the current issues which pose threats to Nurses and other caregivers across the nation, this update would include the following:

None of the caregivers who were arrested and accused of killing their patients were criminally indicted, but Doctor Anna Pou did face a Grand Jury Hearing. It was a terrifying ordeal for her. She was accused of deliberately overdosing patients at Memorial Medical Center and stood to lose her eligibility to practice medicine and possible incarceration. Her advocacy for needed legislative changes associated with protection of caregivers during disasters promoted significant changes in state law.

Many speculated that hospitals were likely to face

litigation. There was intense coverage of the events by the Dallas Morning News, a hometown media organization covering news dealing with the Dallas-based Tenet Healthcare Corp. which had six hospitals in the hurricane stricken area including the Memorial Medical Center. Media focus was riveted on the facility because of the 45 bodies located at the hospital and was the locus of the alleged patient murder crimes. Legal experts posited that jury's would be forced to consider many arcane questions, not the least of which would focus on expected level of preparedness in an area known for its deadly storms. This was the first time **"act of God"** surfaced as a possible defense.

The best retrospective coverage of the Memorial Medical Center disaster saga is found in an article published four years (August, 2009) after that fateful event. Sheri Fink, a physician and staff reporter at ProPublica, in her Pulitzer Prize winning article, **"The Deadly Choices at Memorial"** fully and dramatically captures the angst and collective horror experienced at one hospital during and after Katrina.

Television coverage of the disaster was chaotic, emotional and at times inaccurate. Evacuees from Tulane and Charity hospitals were taken to an airport triage center located at Louis Armstrong International Airport.

According to television reports the facility was operated much like a military field hospital. "The staff was forced to make some difficult decisions about treatment. There are some cases that have come through here where they have to 'black tag' the person, where basically they're just left to die." The lack of any consistency in "sorting/mass casualties or triage" has been the subject of post-Katrina discussions. They range along a priority decision matrix from "healthy pregnant women, premature infants, the gravely ill to those who will likely survive." Experts have identified at least 9 competing models.

The New Katrina Flood: Hospital Liability, a follow-on article by Sheri Fink published January 1, 2010 focused on a lawsuit brought by the family of a patient who died in Pendleton Memorial Methodist Hospital, one of the many New Orleans Healthcare Centers inundated by flood waters during Katrina. She indicated that this lawsuit was uniquely different from previous cases tried under medical malpractice cases where damages are capped at $500,000.

Kristin McMahon, an attorney and chief claims officer for IronHealth, a company that insures hospitals is quoted "This could be a new theory of liability against healthcare institutions — lack of emergency preparedness". The article also quotes Dr. Robert Wise, a vice president of the Joint Commission (TJC) as saying "There are many places that still know they have to move their generators, without power hospitals are literally dead in the water. It's a critical Asset."

We continue: "But most hospitals are juggling multiple priorities and operating on thin margins. Raising generators is not mandatory for hospital accreditation, and government agencies have rarely provided funding for expensive work prior to a disaster. This is a zero sum game now. Who decides it's not important to buy critical machines for the intensive care unit or the operating room versus moving the emergency electrical system?"

"A jury in New Orleans might have an answer," posits Dr. Fink!!!

Well, Yes and No!! Not being a lawyer, I will leave that to others.

Under the headline <u>**"Katrina Lawsuit: Pandora's Box of Hospital Liability"**</u> findlaw.com, using sources from The New York Times and USA Today, discusses what may be a precedent setting case "It was not about medical malpractice — it's about whether or not the hospital's emergency preparedness (or lack thereof) constituted negligence."

The 2007 Louisiana Supreme Court ruling on the death of a ventilator dependent patient cleared the way for the patient's family to seek damages under general liability rather than the damage limiting medical malpractice rule. The family filed for damages in the Orleans Parish Civil District asking for damages in the amount of $11.7 million. The trial started on January 4, 2010 and was settled by the hospital three week later without going to the jury. The records are sealed by the court. A second case went to trial in May of 2010 and again was settled by the hospital prior to going to the jury.

According to Doctor Sheri Fink "more than 100 deaths occurred in New Orleans-area hospitals and nursing homes after Hurricane Katrina...About 200 lawsuits have been filed in Louisiana alleging that these institutions are liable for the deaths and for the suffering of other patients who survived because of corporate failure to plan adequately for flooding and implement evacuation, constituted negligence or medical malpractice.

It appears that the *"Act of God"* defense did not serve the defendants well. Five years after the event it appears that Katrina was a *"God awful storm"* and the Hospital and Healthcare System suffered from Apathy, Denial or Cognitive Dissonance.

Chapter Ten

Lessons Not Learned!

To our Nurses we would say that your noble efforts to influence future workplace safety and security for caregivers is a pledge still unrealized. It takes more than an *apathetic non-federal hospital sector* to leave the trusting public vulnerable to a measurably more hostile environment.

The noble goals of Access, Quality and Affordability have been challenges for decades. Existing national efforts to protect patients from unnecessary death and suffering arising from healthcare acquired infections and treatment errors should be a priority in the nation's health policy. Promoting a healthy insurance system which provides for equitable access to quality care is a just healthcare goal. Reduction of aggregate healthcare costs is critical to any sustained nation-wide provision of healthcare.

Lost in the passionate advocacy for these important

health policy pursuits to bring an acceptable level of care to the nation, is *the reality* that the value of these achievements would pale by comparison in **a multiple Flash-Bang of nuclear or dirty bomb explosions, or slippage of the Pacific/New Madrid seismic plates, or a raging virulent pandemic.**

Hospital and healthcare safety and security functions have morphed into an exclusive clinical domain. We think at a measurable cost to facility safety and security.

Critical Components of the **Public Health and Healthcare** sector have turned a blind eye to the known all-hazards threats to the healthcare workplace or serve as **passive enablers**.

Hospital and healthcare design and construction community has repeatedly ignored the need for more robust and secure built environment. The dual benefits of creating built environments which reduce vulnerabilities to known natural and man-made threats are a "no brainer." As the federal sector and enlightened urban authorities harden their structures it increases the less well protected facilities, making them by definition "soft" targets-targets of opportunity. Design and Construction (D&C) is the "mother of all vulnerability mitigation." AIA, D&C guidance for hospitals and healthcare facilities (2002, 2006,

2010) reflect "business as usual" with little attention given to the need to prepare for known threats (Earthquakes, Floods, Hurricanes, CBRNE error or terror, natural or man-made) to all stakeholders in healthcare. There is little need to discuss the role of design and construction in sustainability of building in disasters. The visual documentation of recent earthquakes and tsunamis across the world leave little chance to trump with the printed word.

Hospital and healthcare human resources community has failed in their duty to provide robust screening policies and procedures in their hiring practices. There are regional differences in compliance with criminal background checks. One state has failed to perform criminal background checks on one-third of their healthcare workforce, even worse, the majority of these employees have close one-on-one contact with the most vulnerable patients within the system. Increased reliance on "outsourced" clinical and administrative personnel without "trust but verify" procedures places the workforce at risk. The loss of central federal registries of healthcare criminal offenders is troublesome. The two-decades old national database of healthcare miscreants is missing. Caregiver criminals have been able to move from state to state with relative ease.

Hospital and healthcare Stewardship — Board and Trustees: Hospital Boards must accept the ultimate responsibility for insuring the safety and security of their institutions. Over the span of a lifetime the culture of Stewardship within the hospital and healthcare industry has changed. The industry has morphed from its altruistic, patient — centered roots into a highly competitive, bottom-line commercial enterprise. That does not mean that the system is not devoid of altruistic, compassionate folks, however, they have limited influence on the industry. Board members come from varied backgrounds. They range from dedicated citizens with little working knowledge of the complexities of hospital administration to highly sophisticated professionals from a number of industries. Many members are drawn from the local communities. Others serve on boards with responsibilities for multiple hospitals located some distance from these organizations. Today's hospital's Boards are focused on the "bottom line" and few have an in-depth exposure to information on all-hazards threats. An important source for their information on this area comes from their administrator and others in the C-suite. As we will see, this subject does not appear to compete well with other issues in C-Suite.

Hospital and healthcare Stewardship — The C-Suite: Hospital Boards hire Administrators to run the day-to-day operations of their organizations. Selection of an administrator is one of the Board's most important duties. Annual surveys (ACHE) of hospital Chief Executive Officers (CEOs) ask this group to prioritize their operational concerns for the past year. Disaster Preparedness did not compete well in the 2010 survey, less than 1% identified all-hazards preparedness as a concern. These are not your run-of-the-mill healthcare executives. They are today's hospital leaders. Patients depend on them to provide for a safe healthcare environment. Employees depend on them to keep them safe from workplace hazards. Investors depend on them for their fiscal stewardship. Board members depend on them to protect their reputations and keep them out of jail. Communities depend on them to make the difference between life and death in times of crisis. In many communities where hospitals are the dominant employers, their future economic existence depends on informed decisions by hospital authorities.

Hospital and healthcare professional all-hazards education: The American College of Healthcare Executives (ACHE) probably the most powerful and influential healthcare executive educational organization in the nation, failed to strongly advocate for all-hazards readiness and opted to let other trade organizations pick up the gauntlet. Failure in early attempts (2004) to attract its membership into all-hazards professional educational programs discouraged any meaningful future offerings. A careful review of educational offerings available from the organization's regional seminars and content of educational offerings available Annual Conferences confirm the lack of advocacy for or deep interest in all-hazards readiness.

Hospital and healthcare Professional media: National healthcare trade media follows the operational concerns of the industry. Heavy coverage of: market share, financial challenges, patient safety and quality (Clinical), personnel shortages, computerized health records, etc. There is considerable interest in hospital design and construction, however, the focus is on patient satisfaction and the issue of facility security is rarely addressed. The most recent articles which deal with "Hospitals of The Future" issues associated with **non-clinical safety and security are essentially ignored.**

Hospital and healthcare Popular Media: Popular magazine media has entered the "cottage Industry" of publishing their list of the best places to receive hospital care for "this or that" condition. They share the same weakness as trade organizations in guiding the trusting public to "best of breed" in quality and safety, in that they fail to assess important dimensions of the locus of care. News coverage of shootings in hospitals often go unchallenged. A recent example is the tragic shooting at Johns Hopkins. Knee-jerk statements of hospital and city authorities border on the absurd, "if you use metal detectors patients will not come, guns in hospitals are not a problem, they are rare, even if you use detectors, patients will circumvent them," etc. The hospital complex has 83 entrances and none of the 400 security force inside the facility is armed. Joint Commission authorities, the hospital's "deeming authority," is back to evaluate "Emergency Management" issues. If faced with a **"Mumbai style attack"** similar to the one experienced by the CAMA hospital in India there would be terrorists within the hospital and no one armed to defend stakeholders. The stage is set for a bloody event.

Hospital and healthcare — external evaluation mechanisms-Emergency Management: The earlier statements by Doctor Robert Wise of the Joint Commission make us question what Accreditation means when it comes to facility safety and security and other issues associated with Emergency Management. If the Joint Commission does not see the need to question emergency generators below the floodplain or 83 entrances to a hospital complex as a potential threat then who does? What if the earlier TJC surveyors noted that emergency generators should be above the floodplain or that 83 entrances to a hospital complex represent a security risk (even for the best hospital in the world) or worse, they did not document the hazards, who will step in to protect the trusting public?

The issue of consumer protection has been with us for some time. Probably best articulated by critics well before the landmark "IOM-To Err is Human." The Presidential Advisory Commission on Consumer Protection's Final Meeting Report, March 1998 captures the essence of the lingering problem in the following quotes: *"Conflicts of interest can arise from multiple sources. For example, private sector accrediting bodies have, as one of their customers, the entities that the organization accredits. The organization to be accredited sometimes is the same organizations that created or fostered the creation of the accrediting entity, and often are necessarily involved in identifying the standards to which they will be held accountable."*

And more to the point, "Quality oversight organizations also have a second set of customers-healthcare consumers — who depend on the work of these organizations to make comparative judgments about the quality of certain types of organizations. This is particularly true when public regulators use accreditation as a means of public standards (e.g., when JCAHO accredited hospitals are deemed to have met Medicare Conditions of Participation) Consumer advocacy organizations become concerned when the accreditation organization seems overly solicitous of the views of the industry, or when very few organizations have their accreditation denied." The 2008 nine month "scoring hiatus" appears to fit this concern.

Hospital and healthcare DHHS oversight: Congress has entrusted direct oversight of the external evaluation process of healthcare facilities to the Center for Medicare and Medicaid Services (CMS). They contract this function to others. If we accept the notion that no one would endorse having emergency generators below the floodplain and Joint Commission experts admit that that situation exists all across the nation, **where does the buck stop?** GAO-04-850, **CMS Needs Additional Authority to Adequately Oversee Patient Safety in Hospitals,**

an annual CMS validation study of JCAHO surveys, released over a year before Katrina, clearly identified the many weaknesses in the these surveys including deficiencies in assessing major **"Environment of Care"** problems which surfaced during Katrina.

Sorry for the following "pain in the acronym," but please stay with me!!!

Hospital and healthcare DHS oversight — FEMA DHS OHA: The Federal Emergency Management Agency (FEMA) in coordination with the Department of Homeland Security, Office of Health Affairs (DHS OHA) have operational responsible for healthcare all-hazards readiness. Under certain circumstances they share that responsibility with the Assistant Secretary for Preparedness and Response (ASPR) in the Department of Health and Human Services. There is one more shared responsibility, Public Health and Healthcare (HPH) National Infrastructure Protection Plan (NIPP). **A hospital which faces the dangers associated with our examples should be of collective concern to everyone in these organizations.**

State and Local Healthcare All-hazards Readiness: State governments are responsible for the health, safety and security of their citizens. For the most part, all hazards events are local. **GAO-10-381T**, released January 25, 2010 contains testimony before the Subcommittee on Management, Investigations, and Oversight Committee on Homeland Security, House of Representatives. It addresses State efforts to plan for medical surge capacity for mass casualty producing events (all-hazards). Some take comfort in the healthcare sector's response to the 9/11 attacks. However, from a healthcare mass casualty perspective, it was a mass mortuary event. Had there been a chemical, biological, radiological attack in tandem with those attacks, the lack of crowd control and porous hospital security **would have resulted in the loss of those facilities for continued care**.

Many state legislative bodies have failed to respond to the need to change existing laws which create barriers to any meaningful healthcare all-hazards response. Oversight of federal grants from DHS and DHHS has been soft. "In brief, we found that the federal government provided funding-guidance and other assistance to help states prepare for medical surge in a mass casualty event. From fiscal years 2002 to 2007, the federal government awarded the states about $2.2 billion through DHHS-ASPR's Hospital Preparedness Program to support activities to meet their preparedness priorities and goals...We cannot report state-specific funding." State level self-reporting for all-hazards compliance without follow-up or confirmation is troubling.

Hospital and healthcare Insurance and Capital Lending Industries: The last of the 2004, 9/11 Commission Recommendations were implemented through P.L. 110-53. One overarching concern expressed by members of the Commission dealt with private sector participation in the national strategy for Homeland Security protection.

"We also encourage the insurance and credit-lending industries to look closely at a company's compliance with (ANSI) standard in assessing its insurability and creditworthiness. We believe that compliance with the standard should define the standard of care owed by a company to its employees and the public for legal purposes. **Private-sector preparedness is not a luxury; it is the cost of doing business in a post 9/11 world.** It is ignored at tremendous potential cost in lives, money, and national security."

We have seen little evidence that the insurance and capital lending organizations meet the spirit of the Commission's recommendation.

Chapter Eleven

The All-Hazards Perfect Storm — Japan, March 2011

As I opened this Chapter, I received a telephone call from a friend asking, "Have you seen the news about the earthquake in Japan?"

There is a certain irony in the timing of this series of events in Japan and a wrap-up of this book. It is an "all-hazards perfect storm," the earthquake, tsunami, nuclear radiation threat and looming biological and epidemic threat posed by avian flu.

The combined reports of avian flu deaths in the region (Indonesia, India, and Bangladesh) and the existence of avian flu infections in Japan's poultry population should be of considerable concern to public health officials.

Post-earthquake/tsunami environments are always a public health nightmare, adding this risk to the mix is horrific.

Since the 1994 Northridge earthquake and its

destructive consequences, the State of California mandated and scheduled its hospital system for seismic upgrading to mitigate the destructive power of future earthquakes. The initial fervor to provide safer workplaces for its healthcare stakeholders quickly cooled and **"to seismically upgrade or not to seismically upgrade hospitals was the question."** For sixteen years it has been a standoff between the Industry and those caregivers who work in those hospitals. It has been difficult to follow the political machinations in years of legislative actions. However, drop-dead dates for implementation of these "mandated" upgrades have come and gone, (through fat and lean economic times). A recent article in the Sacramento Bee leaves one with the impression that the "dust has not settled on the issue" as evidenced by the caption, **"California Hospitals Seek Relief from Seismic Safety Rules."** Over half of the non-federal hospitals in California have not been seismically upgraded and all hospital stakeholders remain at risk in the event of a known greatest hazard to the area (earthquakes). California Nurses Association's pleas for safer workplaces go unanswered.

In the face of the dangers posed by these threats and equally destructive tsunamis, State political authorities continue to "accept the risk" and Congressional and federal agencies sit on the sidelines. Indeed, the principal healthcare advisor (NIAC) for Public Health and Healthcare Sector is the administrator of one of the most prestigious Healthcare systems on the west coast-which the California Nurses Association complain is at great risk to the effects of any earthquake in the area.

The west coast of the United States shares with Japan the "'Ring of Fire' where most quakes occur around the Pacific, where ocean plates constantly shift and plunge. Volcano eruptions, quakes, and tsunamis they generate, threatens millions."

Middle America's **New Madrid Fault** threatens death and destruction from future seismic activity and a cascading Mississippi river tsunami. Lessons learned in Japan from recent costly and deadly earthquakes (1994, 1995, 2004) have created a culture of preparedness and enhanced their capacity to better respond to these events. Robust building codes and retrofitting of built structures have mitigated consequences of urban building collapse.

The earthquake, Tsunami and the companion threat of nuclear plant meltdown and collateral danger to an already suffering population, should act as a heads-up to the United States. Experts remind us that in addition to these naturally occurring disasters there are real threat of radiologic exposures from other forces. The dreaded terrorist nuclear explosion using imported materials or what the 2007 Defense Science Board characterized as "low hanging fruit" and one of the greatest terrorist threat to the nation, unprotected medical use radiological materials, **Cesium 137 (one-half of a dirty bomb)** is found in some 1000 healthcare facilities and research laboratories across the country.

Japan also faces biological, radiologic and chemical threats from protected and unprotected sources in a wide range of research laboratories and other private and government sites. In the United States experts posit that **the greatest biological threats (bio-error/bioterror) come from the escalating number of laboratories** tasked with the mission of finding **countermeasures for biologic agents and toxins expected to be used by terrorists.**

There are lingering concerns over the question of contamination of the greater New Orleans area during and after Katrina. Post Katrina investigators questioned the timeliness of actions taken to safeguard chemical, biological and radiological materials, and additional accounting for infected research animals and other deadly toxins in the **custody of hospitals, healthcare facilities and research entities.**

Chapter Twelve
Final Note

Are We Ready Yet?—Latest Message from your Government—Old Wine in New Bottles, the Solution, Change the Name!!!!

The 2010 publication of a DHHS funded study released by the Center for Biosecurity, University Pittsburg Medical Center "**The Next Challenge in Healthcare Preparedness—Catastrophic Health Events (CHE)**" confirms that the **Public Health and Healthcare** Sector is ill-prepared to deal with large mass casualty producing events.

The 2010 **National Health Security Strategy of the United States of America (NHSS)** is touted as the nation's first National Health Security strategy brings into question the previous twenty years of guidance to the Public Health and Healthcare Sector. **Indeed, it is more like the most recent attempt to reorganize failed attempts to** achieve some level of Homeland Security healthcare readiness.

A final note to the **"Nurses in Hell Group,"** If past is prologue, it tells us that Americans are reluctant to prepare for known or perceived existential threats. This propensity for **"reactive"** rather than **"proactive"** is alive and well in the hearts and minds of those who lead the provision of healthcare to today's trusting public.

What else could the public expect from an industry where **"an ounce of prevention is worth a pound of cure"** falls on hearing-challenged ears? Prevention over intervention rings true, however, and **at the end of the day the more profitable intervention trumps the more valuable course of prevention every time.**

P.S. Recent headlines provide little encouragement that the Hospital industry "gets it" —
- "Cal Pacific, Stanford hope to postpone huge seismic upgrades"
- "U. S. still unprepared for threats, 9-11 Commission chiefs say"
- "Americans Doubt Feds in Disaster Management"
- "Special Needs Require Special Preparedness"

FINAL NOTE

- "Emergency Readiness Said Lacking at U.S. Nuclear Sites"
- "$1b effort yields no bioterror defenses"
- "National database riddled with holes: Records missing on disciplined healthcare workers"
- "Bioterrorism's Threat Persists as Top Security Risk"
- "New Hospital Industry Bid to Duck Earthquake Safety Deadlines to Put More Patients at Risk"
- "Quake rolls across Baja"
- "U. S. sees homegrown Muslim extremism as rising threat: This may have been the most dangerous year since 9/11, anti-terrorism experts say"
- "W.Pa. bioterrorism lab fails inspection"
- "FBI: 100 Percent Chance of WMD Attack"
- "Small terror groups are homeland challenge of future — Intel chief: Spy agencies can prevent a Sept. 11-style attack, but smaller attacks will be harder"
- "Workers Imperiled by Lack of Pandemic Flu Readiness"
- "Nuclear Waste Piles Up at Hospitals"
- "Dirty Bomb Recovery Plans Lacking"
- "The Little Nukes That Got Away"

Shadowing those headlines are *Headlines* that indicate that there are consequences for failure to prepare for and respond to, known all-hazards events. "Just in time" for a "Black Swan Event" (Fukoshima, Japan) to remind the trusting public that the threats are real.

- "Katrina Lawsuit: Pandora's Box of Hospital Liability"
- "Katrina negligence lawsuit has implications for all hospitals"
- "The New Katrina Flood: Hospital Liability"
- "Weighing the cost of disaster-Trial could raise stakes for emergency planning"
- "U. S. Thinks of Strategy for the Unthinkable."

"The wheels of justice grind slowly and exceedingly fine."
–Anonymous

"The history of man is a graveyard of great cultures that came to catastrophic ends because of their incapacity for planning rational, voluntary reaction to change."
–Eric Fromm

Appendices A – D

APPENDIX A
University of Tennessee College of Nursing
INFORMED CONSENT STATEMENT—TO BE
READ TO PARTICIPANT

I. **INTRODUCTION OF THE RESEARCHER**

   My name is Marti Jordan-Welch and I am the nurse researcher for this study. I am presently working to complete my doctorate in nursing from The University of Tennessee in Knoxville. This research is in fulfillment of requirements for my doctorate. I also have a masters degree in nursing, and have worked for 23 years in nursing.

   1. Do you have any questions about me or my background? ☐ Yes ☐ No

II. **TO BEGIN THIS INTERVIEW AND TO PROTECT YOUR CONFIDENTIALITY, I AM ASKING YOU TO CHOOSE A PSEUDONYM.**

   Please state the pseudonym you have selected for yourself and today's date. (Pause)

III. **DIGITAL RECORDING**

   This study is "An existential phenomenological study of the lived experience of providing nursing care during and after Hurricane Katrina" and our interview will be digitally recorded.

1. Do you understand that in order to protect your confidentiality this consent is being digitally recorded and no signatures will be obtained from you?   ☐ Yes   ☐ No

The next sections give you information about what you can expect when you participate.

IV. INTRODUCTION OF THE RESEARCH

You are being invited to participate in a research study being conducted by me. The purpose of this study is to explore and describe the experience of providing nursing care to patients in acute or long-term care facilities in the Gulf Coast Region, Southern Louisiana, or Southern Mississippi during and immediately after Hurricane Katrina (from August 28, 2005 through September 12, 2005).

1. Is this clear to you?   ☐ Yes   ☐ No

2. Do you have any questions about the purpose of the study?   ☐ Yes   ☐ No

V. INFORMATION ABOUT PARTICIPANT'S INVOLVEMENT IN THE STUDY

1. Do you understand that in this study you will be asked to talk with me face to face about this experience? Most interviews will probably last about an hour. The exact time that you will speak with me will be decided by you. If you are finished with all you need or want to say in less than 1 hour, that is fine. If it takes longer than an hour, that will also be fine with me. Do you have any questions about the length of the interview?   ☐ Yes   ☐ No

2. If necessary, the interview can be stopped, split, and/or reconvened. Do you understand that you can request that the interview be split, reconvened for a second interview, or stopped entirely at any time?   ☐ Yes   ☐ No

3. The information obtained during this study may be

published in a professional journal or presented at a professional meeting. When this information is presented at conferences or published, it will be presented either as group findings, or without personal identifiers linked to you. You will not be linked to any information in any way. Your identity will not be revealed to anyone.

Do you have any questions about how your identity will be protected? ☐ Yes ☐ No

The next sections give you information about the risks and benefits of participating in this study.

VI. RISKS & PROTECTIONS

In this study, the physical risks are minimal, meaning that they are no greater than you would experience by talking to anyone in everyday life.

However, one possible risk could be emotional distress. As you think about the experience, you may become emotionally upset by recalling your hurricane experience. If you are already experiencing psychological problems, you may not want to participate. If you do choose to participate, the interview may be stopped either by you or by me if your stress seems too great.

1. If you have any questions about whether you should participate or not, please let me know now, or ask to discuss it at this time. _____Yes _____No If you decide you want to talk about this at any other time, please stop me and we will talk about it then. Do you understand and agree? ☐ Yes ☐ No

There have been some news reports that nurses have gotten into trouble with their employers for talking to researchers, or with the authorities about their activities during the hurricane. Because of these reports, some people who participate in this study might worry about their jobs or licenses, or about being reported to the authorities.

To help put you at ease, and to reduce your risk as much as possible, I am collecting minimal information about you, and recording this consent rather than having you sign any documents. That is also why you are using a pseudonym. Most important, I am asking that if you participated in any illegal activity during the course of your practice, or saw or participated in anything that you worry might be illegal or unethical, you do not discuss it with me. Instead, if you participated in anything illegal, or worry that something you did or saw was unethical, and want to discuss it with someone, you should seek out the advice of a trained counselor or attorney. If you discuss illegal activity with me, I am obligated by law to report those acts to the authorities.

2. Do you understand that I am asking you to limit your discussions to your experience of giving nursing care during Hurricane Katrina—excluding any actions which were against the law? ☐ Yes ☐ No

3. If you participated in actions that were against the law or unethical, and wish to discuss them with someone who can help you, you should seek the advice of legal counsel. Do you understand that? ☐ Yes ☐ No

4. You are free to discuss any other aspect of your experience of providing care during Hurricane Katrina. You can discuss your feelings, the meaning of the experience, or anything else that you would care to reveal. Do you understand the kinds of information that I am looking for? ☐ Yes ☐ No

5. Do you have any questions about what this study is about, or the things that we can discuss? If so, I can talk to you more about this now. During this study, I will know you by first name only. I will only collect information about your age, gender, educational level, and years as a nurse. I have asked you to pick a pseudonym and I will record this consent with that name and refer to you by that name only during the interview. When you are referring to your place of employment, refer to the place by "Hospital A" or "Hospital B", to doctors the same, and to co-workers by first name only. When the interviews are transcribed, your pseudonym will be changed to another

pseudonym. After the study is completed I will destroy your contact information.

6. Do you understand that I will not release this information to anyone, except as required by law? ☐ Yes ☐ No
7. Do you have any questions about the risks or protections of this study? ☐ Yes ☐ No

VII. BENEFITS

The benefits of this study are that you will be able to talk to a caring professional, me, about what it was like providing nursing care during and immediately after Hurricane Katrina without the risk of judgment. This research interview holds the potential to be cleansing and healing. You may provide critical information that might help nurses better understand what it was like providing care during and immediately after Hurricane Katrina and prepare those who work in the Gulf Coast Region during hurricanes in the future. You may also help nurse educators better understand this experience so that they can provide education to future nurses, which may help them cope with these situations in the future. A better understanding of this experience may also help nursing administrators to develop policies that help nurses address situations like this.

1. Is this clear to you? ☐ Yes ☐ No
2. Do you have any questions about the benefits of this study? ☐ Yes ☐ No

VIII. CONFIDENTIALITY

In addition to all the other things I have told you about protection, the information in this study will be kept confidential. Interviews will be transcribed by me or a transcriptionist who has signed a confidentiality pledge. Transcriptions will be read by my dissertation committee and the Interpretive Phenomenology Group which meets weekly at the UT College of Nursing; they have also signed a confidentiality pledge. This group is made up of other researchers who will help assure that I understand the data accurately. The data from the interviews will be entered into a file on my computer and will be protected by a password. The digital recordings will be transferred to a CD. The CD's and copies of the transcripts will be stored at my office in a locked file. The contact information and the CD's will be destroyed after the study is complete. No reference will be made to you in oral or written reports which could link you to this study.

1. Is this clear to you?   ☐ Yes   ☐ No
2. Do you have any questions about confidentiality?   ☐ Yes   ☐ No

IX. COMPENSATION

You will not be paid for participating in this study.

1. Do you agree to this interview, knowing that you will not be paid for your time?   ☐ Yes   ☐ No
2. If you have any questions about this, we can discuss it now.

X. EMERGENCY MEDICAL TREATMENT

The University of Tennessee does not "automatically" reimburse you for medical claims or other compensation. If physical injury is suffered in the course of the research, or for more information, please notify the investigator in charge, me, Marti Jordan-Welch, at my office (601) 266-6950.

1. Do you understand that The University of Tennessee does not automatically reimburse medical claims?   ☐ Yes   ☐ No

While we will not pay for your medical claims, you will be given a list of mental health providers if you suffer emotional distress during the study, or if you request it. To the extent possible, this list will be of providers who are currently in practice in the Gulf region. It will also include crisis "hot lines". It would be your responsibility to contact these providers and make your own arrangements for care, including your own arrangements for payment.

2. Is this clear to you? ___ Yes ___ No
3. Do you understand the information about emergency medical treatment? ☐ Yes ☐ No

You may also stop the interview at anytime if you are becoming emotionally distressed, fatigued, or decide not to continue. A second interview can be scheduled at your convenience if you wish to continue this interview over to another session for any reason.

4. Is it clear that you have the opportunity to stop the interview at any time, split the interview, or reconvene it at another time? ☐ Yes ☐ No

XI. CONTACT INFORMATION

If you have any questions about the study or the procedures, (or if you experience adverse effects as a result of participating in this study), you may contact the researcher, me, Marti Jordan-Welch at work: 118 College Drive #5095, Hattiesburg, MS 39406, or (601) 266-6950. If you have any questions about your rights as a participant, contact the Office of Research Compliance Officer at The University of Tennessee, (865) 974-3466.

Is this clear to you? ☐ Yes ☐ No

XII. VOLUNTARY PARTICIPATION

Participation in this study is voluntary; you may decline to participate without penalty. If the decision is made to participate, you may withdraw from this study at any time without penalty and without loss of benefits to which you are otherwise entitled. If you withdraw from the study before the interview is completed, you may choose to have your interview information destroyed.

Is this clear to you? ☐ Yes ☐ No

XIII. CONSENT

Now that all this information has been given to you do you have any remaining questions? ☐ Yes ☐ No

Do you agree to participate in this study? ☐ Yes ☐ No

Please re-state your pseudonym and the date.

Consent given verbally and digitally recorded ☐

Date: _____

Investigator's signature _____

Date: _____

APPENDIX B
TRANSCRIBER'S PLEDGE OF CONFIDENTIALITY

As a transcribing typist of this research project, "A phenomenological study of the lived experience of registered nurses caring for patients during and after Hurricane Katrina", I understand that I will be hearing digital recordings of confidential interviews. The information on these recordings has been revealed by research participants who participated in this project on good faith that their interviews would remain strictly confidential. I understand that I have a responsibility to honor this confidentially agreement. I hereby agree not to share any information on these recordings with anyone except the primary researcher of this project. Any violation of this agreement would constitute a serious breach of ethical standards, and I pledge not to do so.

Transcribing Typist _____

Date: _____

APPENDIX C

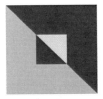

REGISTERED NURSES
Want to tell your story?

Marti Jordan-Welch MSN, RN, Nurse Researcher

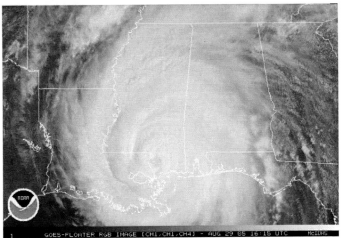

Were you a Registered Nurse caring for patients in a hospital the day of Hurricane Katrina and in the days after it? Would you like to talk about what it was like caring for those patients during the hurricane. A nurse researcher from Hattiesburg will be conducting a study to find out what it was like caring for patients during and after Hurricane Katrina.

Findings from this study may help nurses be better prepared to handle an experience like this in the future.

Information will be kept confidential.

Please contact me by phone,
e-mail, or regular mail
Marti Jordan-Welch
118 College Drive #5095
Hattiesburg, MS 39406

Phone: (601) 266-6950

To protect your confidentiality when you call, please leave only your first name and phone number.

Email: marti.jordan60@comcast.net

APPENDIX D
RESEARCH TEAM MEMBER'S PLEDGE OF CONFIDENTIALITY

As a member of this project's research team, "A phenomenological study of the lived experience of registered nurses caring for patients during and after Hurricane Katrina", I understand that I will be reading transcriptions of confidential interviews. The information in these transcripts has been revealed by research participants who participated in this project on good faith that their interviews would remain strictly confidential. I understand that I have a responsibility to honor this confidentially agreement. I hereby agree not to share any information in these transcriptions with anyone except the primary researcher of this project, his/her doctoral chair, or other members of this research team. Any violation of this agreement would constitute a serious breach of ethical standards, and I pledge not to do so.

Research Team Member _____

Date: _____

References

Recent Author Publications that pertain to Homeland Security CBRNE and All-Hazards Healthcare Readiness

Blair, J.D., **All-Hazards "HVA" for Non-Federal Healthcare CBRNE Readiness: A Level Playing Field?** Inside Homeland Security, Volume 3, Issue 5, Sept/Oct 2005.

Blair, J.D., **Homeland Security and the Non-Federal Healthcare Sector: Evaluation of Your Incident Command System (ICS),** Journal of Healthcare Protection Management, Volume 21, Number 2, Summer 2005.

Blair, J.D., **Homeland Security and Non-Federal Health Sector: Incident Command Structure.** Hospital Fire Marshal's News (HFMA), April 2005.

Blair, J.D., **National Response Plan and the Non-Federal Healthcare Industry's Design and Construction Community,** Matrix, 2005.

Blair, J.D., **Healthcare Readiness for CBRNE Terrorist Events, Emergency Response Manual, Chapter 25,** Anti-Terrorism Board Certified Anti-Terrorism Specialist (ATAB).

Blair, J.D., Edwards, J. T., **Critical Issues for Homeland Security and Healthcare Readiness,** Journal of Healthcare Risk Management, October 2005.

Blair, J.D., **Is Healthcare the Weak Link in the Homeland Security Chain?** Medical News, January 2006, KY Medical News (KY, IN, OH).

Blair, J.D., **Homeland Security and the Non-Federal Sector Readiness.** Hospital Fire Marshal's Association, Part 1, December 2005, Part 2, January 2006.

Blair, J.D., **Perspectives on Advanced Directives, Monograph,** Task Force Member, American Society for Healthcare Risk Management, August 2006.

Blair, J.D., **Is The Healthcare Industry Prepared for Terrorism?** Journal of Healthcare Protection Management, Volume 22, Number 1.

Blair, J.D., Silver, R. B., Modern Healthcare, **"Commentary"** Daily Dose and Modern Healthcare Online, January 2007.

Blair, J.D., Scanlon, P. A., **Pandemic Flu Threat and Business Continuity.** Elliot Consulting Group, News Letter.

Blair, J.D., Dluzneski, P.K., **Evolving Roles and Responsibilities for Healthcare Security Professionals: The Non-Federal Healthcare Sector Meets NIMS and NIPP,** Journal of Healthcare Protection Management, January 2007.

Blair, J.D., **NIPPS vs. Non-Federal Hospital Design and Construction,** Letter to the Editor, Health Affairs, July 2006.

Blair, J.D., **Lagging Healthcare Sector,"** Updates and Responses, HSToday.us, April 2007.

REFERENCES

Blair, J.D., **"Are Medical Facilities Doing Enough to Prepare for Catastrophic Events?"** Healthcare Construction and Operation, March 2008.

Blair, J.D., Scanlon, P. A., **Reflections on a "Motto,"** Hospital Fire Marshals Association, HFMA NEWS, September 2008.

Blair, J.D., Scanlon, P. A., Dluzneski, P.D., **To Protect in Place or Evacuate? That is the Question,** Journal of Health Protection Management, Volume 24, Number 2, September 2008.

Blair, J.D., **Is the Healthcare Industry Prepared for Terrorism?** Revisited, Inside Homeland Security, Volume 7, Issue 1, Spring 2009.

Blair, J.D., **GITMO Detainees and U.S. Host Communities: Is Your Hospital Prepared to Live with Terrorist Inmates in Your Backyard?** Journal of Healthcare Protection Management, Volume 25, Number 2, Summer 2009.

Blair, J.D., **GITMO Detainees and U.S. Host Communities: Is Your Hospital Prepared to Live with Terrorist Inmates in Your Backyard?** Inside Homeland Security, Volume 7, Issue 4, Winter 2009.

Blair, J.D., **James D. Blair On What Hospitals Can Do To Overcome Deficiencies in All-Hazards Preparedness, IAHSS Directions,** Volume 21, Number 3, 2008 Journal.

Book

UNREADY: To Err is Human — The Other Neglected Side of Hospital Safety and Security, Amazon, Paper and Kindle, July 2010.

Author References—Family Security Matters (FSM) Series

Blair, J.D., **Bio Threats, Bioterror and Bioerror,** FSM, October 16, 2010

Blair, J.D., **Terrorists On the Move With New Flexibility in Target Size and Selection,** FSM, October 27, 2010

Blair, J.D., **Vigilance is Necessary for Traditional Domestic "Anti-Groups,** FSM, November 4, 2010

Blair, J. D., **Implementation of Security Recommendations Delayed and Confused,** FSM, November 12, 2010

Blair, J.D., **An Old Soldier Looks at The Fort Hood Killings,** FSM, November 16, 2010

Blair, J.D., **Is Enough Being Done to Ensure Hospitals are Safe From Terrorist or Criminal Attacks?** FSM, December 18, 2010

Blair, J.D., **Hospital Stewardship and the Culture of Preparedness-1,** FSM, December 22, 2010

Blair, J. D., **Hospital Stewardship and the Culture of Preparedness-2,** FSM, December 31, 2010

Blair, J.D., **Hospital Emergency Preparedness-1: To the Rear March,** FSM, January 21, 2011

Blair, J.D., **Hospital Emergency Management Oversight,** FSM, January 26, 2011

Blair, J.D., **Hospital Emergency Preparedness: Are We There Yet?** FSM, February 3, 2011

REFERENCES

Author References — Examiner.com, Washington D.C. Public Health and Healthcare Expert

Blair, J.D., **The Terrorist Attack Which Brought Russia to its Knees,** December 7, 2009

Blair, J.D., **GITMO Detainees to Rural Mid-America — Illinois Bound?** December 10, 2009

Blair, J.D., **Mammography and Pap Smears,** November 24, 2009

Blair, J.D., **Taps for Direct Healthcare for Military Retirees: The Slippery Slope,** November 21, 2009

Blair, J.D., **NOT IN MY BACKYARD: GITMO DETAINEES TO U.S.; MORE THAN "NO INMATE HAS ESCAPED YET" ISSUE,** November 15, 2009

Blair, J.D., **You Think the Military Healthcare System has Security Problems,** November 11, 2009

Blair, J.D., **Fort Hood-Terrorism's Cascading Effect,** November 11, 2009

Blair, J.D., **Who Treats the Healthcare and Security Community?** November 9, 2009

Blair, J.D., **Welcome HIV/AIDS-Land of Liberty-Obama Ends US Travel Ban On Visitors, Immigrants With HIV/AIDS,** November 1, 2009

Blair, J.D., **"So It Will Never Happen Again,"** October 28, 2009

Blair, J.D., **H1N1-The Horrors of Benign or Not So Benign Neglect,** October 25, 2009

Blair, J.D., **H1N1 VS Bioterrorism,** October 22, 2009

Blair, J.D., **What Ever Happened to the 9/11 Commission Recommendations on Private Sector Readiness?** October 21, 2009

Blair, J.D., **The Late Senate Healthcare Lion, A Lamb on Homeland Security,** October 21, 2009

Blair, J.D., **Time for Healthcare Reform: Congressional Oversight?** October 18, 2009

Blair, J.D., **Time for Healthcare Reform: Accreditation?** October 18, 2009

Blair, J.D., **Time for Healthcare Reform: Greed and Corruption Blind Spot,** October 12, 2009

Blair J.D., **Time for Healthcare Risk Oversight Blind Spot-1,** October 9, 2009

Blair, J.D., **Your Health-The Life you Save May be Your Own,** October 6, 2009

Blair, J.D., **Time for Healthcare Reform: Victim of Bait and Switch,** September 30, 2009

Blair, J.D., **Time for Healthcare Reform: Hospital Accreditation, Blind Spot, Blinders or Worse,** September 28, 2009

Blair, J.D., **Time for Healthcare Reform: To Protect or not Protect, is half a loaf better than none?** September 21, 2009

Blair, J.D., **Time for Healthcare Reform: Cesium-137 and Dirty Bombs- 2, Is your Hospitals safe?** September 22, 2009

Blair, J.D., **Time for Healthcare Reform-"Low hanging fruit" ½ of the mix for the dreaded terrorist "Dirty Bomb.,"** September 21, 2009

REFERENCES

Blair, J.D., **Time for Healthcare Reform: Part 1, It begins with Design and Construction,** September 18, 2009

Blair, J.D., **Time for Healthcare Reform: What is being overlooked?** September 18, 2009

Blair, J.D., H1N1 **Swine Flu and other Calamities: State and Local Prisons/Jail Inmates,** September 18, 2009

Blair, J.D., H1N1 **Swine Flu: Federal Prisoners Competing for Limited Community Resources,** September 13, 2009

Blair, J.D., H1N1 **Swine Flu Treatment Priorities: Kicking Grandma off the Ventilator,** September 13, 2009

Blair, J.D., H1N1 **Children at Risk: Kids are not Miniature Adults,** September 9, 2009

Blair, J.D., **Pandemic Flu: What did four years and billions of dollars get us?** September 9, 2009

Guide to Emergency Management and Related Terms, Definitions, Concepts, Acronyms, Organisms, Programs, Guidance and Legislation, B. Wayne Blanchard, Ph.D., CEM, January 22, 2008 (Date of Last Modification)

The U.S. Government Accountability Office (GAO) is an independent, nonpartisan agency that works for Congress. Often called the "congressional watchdog," GAO investigates how the federal government spends taxpayer dollars. The GAO responds to requests from Congress and their products back to the Congress to answer specific questions asked by the body. As you will see in the GAO Reports, they have dutifully reported on requested areas of investigation. The scope of the GAO's investigations is limited to carefully worded requests. GAO contacts explain that resources also serve as a barrier to more comprehensive coverage of issues. Specific reports include:

2002

GAO-02-141T — Bioterrorism: Public Health and Medical Preparedness

GAO-02-150T — Homeland Security: Key Elements to Risk Management

2003

GAO-03-101 — Major Management Challenges and Program Risks...

GAO-03-233 — Critical Infrastructure: Challenges for Selected Agencies and...

GAO-03-924 — Hospital Preparedness: Most Urban Hospitals Have...

REFERENCES

2004

GAO-04-360R — HHS Bioterrorism Preparedness: States...

GAO-04-458T — Public Health Preparedness: Response Capacity Improving...

GAO-04-850 — Medicare: CMS Needs Additional Authority to Adequately...

2005

GAO-05-1053T — Hurricane Katrina: Providing Oversight of the Nation's Pre...

2006

GAO-06-365R — Preliminary Observations on Hurricane Response..

GAO-06-443R — Evacuation of Hospitals and Nursing Homes...

GA0-06-576R — Status of the Health care System in New Orleans...

GAO-06-618 — Catastrophic Disaster: Enhanced Leadership Capabilities...

GAO-06-826 — Disaster Preparedness: Limitations in Federal Evacuation...

GAO-06-870 — National Emergency Powers

GAO-06-1003 — Status of Hospital and Emergency Department in Greater...

2007

GA0-07-39 — Critical Infrastructure Protection: Progress Coordinating Government

GAO-07-395T — Homeland Security: Preparing for and Responding to Disasters

GAO-07-706R — Critical Infrastructure: Sector Plans and Sector Council Continue...

GAO-07-833T — Homeland Security: Management and Programmatic Challenges

GAO-07-1142T — Homeland Security: Observations on DHS and FEMA Efforts...

2008

GAO-08-36 — Influenza Pandemic: Opportunities Exist to Address Critical...

GAO-08-369 — Natural Disaster Response: FEMA should take action to Improve...

GAO-08-539 — Influenza Pandemic: Federal Agencies Should Continue to assist...

GAO-08-610 — September 11: HHS Needs to Develop a Plan that Incorporates...

GAO-08-668 — Emergency Preparedness: States are Planning for Medical Surge...

GAO-08-768 — National Response Framework: FEMA Needs Policies and...

GAO-O8-808 — Healthcare associated Infections in Hospitals: An Overview...

GAO-08-RL34585 — The Emergency Management Assistance Compact...

REFERENCES

2009

GAO-09-563 — Hurricane Katrina Barriers to Mental Health Service...

GAO-09-651 — Urban Area Security Initiative: FEMA Lacks Measures to...

GAO-09-909T — Influenza Pandemic: Gaps in Pandemic Planning and Preparedness

2010

GAO-10-60 — Center for Medicare and Medicaid Services: Deficiencies in Contract

GAO-10-73 — Influenza Pandemic: Monitoring and Assessing the Status of the...

GAO-10-381 — Emergency Preparedness: State Efforts to Plan for Medical surge...

GAO-10-610 — September 11: HHS Needs to Develop a Plan that Incorporates...

The Congressional Research Service (CRS) serves shared staff to congressional committees and Members of Congress. CRS experts assist at every stage of the legislative process — from the early considerations that precede bill drafting, through committee hearings and floor debate, to the oversight of enacted laws and various agency activities. Reference documents include:

CRS-R40159, Public Health and Medical Preparedness and Response: Issues...

CRS-R40246, DHS Assistance to the States and Localities: Summary and Issues...

CRS-R40418, Oversight of High-Containment Biological Labs...

CRS-R40554, The 2009 Influenza Pandemic: An Overview...

CRS-R41080, The National Commission on Children and Disasters:

CRS-R41646, Public Health and Medical Emergency Management: Issues 112...

CRS-RI33579, The Public Health and Medical Response: Issues for 111...

CRS-RI33589, The Pandemic and All-Hazards Preparedness Act...

CRS-RI33738, Gulf Coast Hurricanes: Addressing Survivors...

CRS-RI34758, The National Response Framework: Overview...

CRS-RL31225, Bioterrorism: Summary of CRS/National Health Policy...

REFERENCES

CRS-RL34724, Would an Influenza Pandemic Quality as a Major Disaster...

CRS-RL40159, Bioterrorism: Federal Efforts to Address...

CRS-RS22254, The Americans with Disabilities Act and Emergency...

CRS-RS22602, Public Health Preparedness and Response: Issues 110...

CRS-RS22840, Organizing for Homeland Security...

Non-Author Books

Jordan, M., P.h.D., *Nursing in Hell: The Katrina Experience,* Lambert Academic Publishing, November, 2009.

Joint Commission Resources, *Getting the Board on Board: What Your Board Needs to Know About Quality and Patient Safety,* 2007.

Ramsey, D. A., Rush, J., *Unprepared,* Daydreamer Books, 2010.

Diaz, T., Newman, B., *Lightning Out of Lebanon: Hezbollah Terrorists on American Soil,* Ballantine Books, 2005.

Natural Disasters: *Protecting the Public's Health,* Pan American Health Organization, Scientific Publication No-575.

Management of Dead Bodies after Disasters, Field Manual 2006.

Health Care Facilities Handbook, NFPA 99, 2005 Edition.

Nuclear Radiation Does Not Make You Glow, Prepared by Ecology and Environment, Include., and The Palladino Company, Inc, U. S. Environmental Protection Agency Emergency Response Section, Region 9, 2007.

Humanitarian Supply Management and Logistics in the Health Sector, Pan American Health Organization 2001.

OSHA Reference Guide, *What You Need to Know in Healthcare,* HCPro, Inc., 2004.

American Board for Certification in Homeland Security, Copy National Response Framework, January 2009.

Dorin, A. F., *Jihad and American Medicine,* Praeger Security International, November 2008.

Gabriel, B., *They Must Be Stopped,* St. Martin's Press, N.Y., September 2008.

Gingrich, N., Pavey, D., Woodbury, A., *Saving Lives & Saving Money,* Gingrich Communications, Inc., 2003.

Non-Author Articles

"FBI, nuclear agency investigates terrorism suspect," *CNN.com,* March 12, 2010.

Adcox, S., "Nuclear Waste Piles Up at Hospitals," *Associated Press,* September 26, 2008.

ADVISEN, "Bill would block hospitals' hiring of own inspectors: Legislator says conflict of interest endangers public safety," *hcfpn.advisen.com,* April 08, 2008.

ADVISEN, "Earthquake risk-Tales of the Unexpected T1 Forget Hurricane, Reinsurers Fear a Monster Earthquake," *advisen.com,* September 03, 2008.

Ali Zulfigar., King, L., "Pakistan's Taliban Leader threatens attacks in the U.S.," *L.A. Times,* April 2009.

REFERENCES

Arquilla, J., "U.S. not ready for Mumbai-like terror attack, *sfgate.com*, November 21, 2010.

Associated Press Release, "W.Pa. bioterrorism lab fails inspection," AP, August 26, 2009.

Associated Press: "Study: Terrorists shifting focus to 'soft' targets," *STRATFOR.com* report, September 8, 2009.

Baldor, L., "Small Terror Groups are Homeland Challenge of Future," *Homeland1.com*, April 2010.

Balwin, T., Ramaprasad, S., Dsmda, M., "Understanding Public confidence in Government to prevent Terrorist Attacks," *Journal of Homeland Security and Emergency Management*, Volume 5, Issue 1, Article 4, 2008.

Barrow, B., "Katrina recovery review ordered by new FEMA leader," *nola.com*, January 28, 2009.

Bender, B., "$1b effort yields no bioterror defenses" *boston.com*, January 17, 2011.

Bender, B., "Security specialists say U.S. is more vulnerable to attack," *Boston.com*, September 11, 2008.

Blesch, G., "Hospital Settles in Katrina-Related Case," *Modern Healthcare*, January 27, 2010.

Blesh, G., "Weighing the cost of disaster, Trial could raise stakes for emergency planning, *Modern Healthcare*, Legal, January 25, 2010.

Blumenthal, L., "Earthquake fault much larger, more dangerous than thought" *mclachyde.com*, May 22, 2009.

Bowman, D., "National database riddled with holes: Records on disciplined healthcare workers" *fiercehealthcare.com*, February 17, 2010.

Brownlee, K., "New Orleans and Efficient Proximate Cause" *Claims Magazine,* September. 2006.

Burby, R., "Hurricane Katrina and the Paradoxes of Government Disaster Policy: Bring About Wise Government Decisions for Hazardous Areas," *ann.sagepub.com,* October, 2006.

Burton, L., "The Constitutional Roots of All-Hazards Policy, Management, and Law," *The Berkeley Electronic Press,* bepress.com, 2008.

California Nurses Association, "Many Hospitals Are Not Ready for H1N1: Nurse Survey Shows Deficiencies in Hospital Swine Flu Readiness," *calnurses.org,* August 2009.

CDC Center for Disease Control and Prevention H1N1 Flu, "Interim Guidance for Correctional and Detention Facilities on Novel Influenza A (H1N1) Virus," *CDC.gov,* May 24, 2009.

Chambers, H., "Construction: 8 Complexes are Unsafe, According to State," *San Diego Business Journal,* April 19, 2010.

Chan, S., Harris, G., "Hurricane and Floods Overwhelmed Hospitals," *nytimes.com,* September 14, 2005.

Clark, C., "10 Years after To Err is Human: Are Hospitals Safer?" *HealthLeaders Media,* November 2009.

CNN, "Evacuations resume at flooded hospital," *cnnworldnews,* September 2, 2005.

Douglas, W., "U.S. still unprepared for threats, 9-11 Commission chiefs say," *miamiherald.com,* March 03, 2011.

Elzer, R. M., "Guide to CMS Compliance," *Journal of Healthcare Management,* Volume 55, Number 2, March/April 2010.

REFERENCES

Ephron, D., Hosenball, M., "Recruited for Jihad? About 20 Young Somali-American Men in Minneapolis Have Recently Vanished," *Newsweek*, February 2, 2009.

FEMA, "Closely Monitoring Midwest Earthquake and Aftershocks," *fema.gov*, April 08, 2008.

FEMA, "NIMS Alert: FY 2008 and 2009 NIMS Implementation Objectives for Healthcare Organizations," *fema.gov*, June 2008.

FEMA, "NIMS Alert: The National Preparedness Directorate Release of Public Health and Medical Resource Typing Definitions and Job Titles," *fema.gov*, January 2009.

FEMA, Hurricane Pam Exercise Concludes, R6-4-093, July 23, 2004.

Fink, S., "Deadly Choices at Memorial," *propublica.org*, August 27, 2009.

Fink, S., "Lawsuit Against New Orleans Hospital Settles Shortly After Trial Begins," *propublica.org*, March 23, 2011.

Fink, S., "Lessons for Hospitals from Hurricane Gustav" *huffingtonpost.com*, September 1, 2008

Fink, S., "State Follows Up on Our Katrina Hospital Investigation — and We Follow Up Too," *proreplica.com*, September 4, 2009.

Fink, S., "The New Katrina Flood: Hospital Liability," *newyorktimes.com*, January 1, 2010.

Fink, S., "Trial to Open in Lawsuit Connected to Hospital Deaths After Katrina," *propublica.org*, March 20, 2011.

Fink, S., "U.S. Health Care System Unprepared for Major Nuclear Emergency," *propublica.org*, April 7, 2011.

Flanagan, B., Gregory, E., Hallisey E., Heitgerd, J., Lewis, B., "A Social Vulnerability Index for Disaster Management," *Journal of Homeland Security and Emergency Management*, Volume 8, Issue 1, Article 3, 2011.

Friedman R., Cannon, W. "Homeland Security and Community Policing: Competing Public Safety Policies," *Journal of Homeland Security and Emergency Management*, Volume 4, Issue 4, Article 2, 2007.

Gabriel, B., "The Enemy Next Door: Terrorists Among Us," *Inside Homeland Security*, Volume 7, Issue 4, Winter 2009.

Gacki-Smith, J., Juarez, A. M., Boyett, L., Homeyer, C., Robinson, L., MacLean, S. L., "Violence Against Nurses Working in U.S. Emergency Departments," *Journal of Healthcare Protection Management*, Volume 26, 2010;26(1):81-99.

Gaynor, M., "Have the Katrina lessons been learned?," *renewamerica.us*, August 27, 2008

Gorman, S., "Bioterrorism's Threat Persists As Top Security Risk," *Wall Street Journal*, August 4, 2008.

Gorman, S., "Terror Threat More Diverse, Study Says" *wsj.com*, September 10, 2010.

Griffin, D., Johnson, K., "Report probes New Orleans hospital deaths," *CNN.com*, January, 2008.

Hall, M., "Now Labeled a Pandemic, Swine Flu Poses Threat to Healthcare Workers," *AFL-CIO NOW Blog*, June 12, 2009.

Hays, D., "D&O Rates Seen Headed For The Outer Planets," *propertyandcasualtyinsurancenews.com*, April 10, 2008.

REFERENCES

Hays, J., Ebinger C. "The Private Sector and the Role of Risk and responsibility in securing the Nation's Infrastructure," *Journal of Homeland Security and Emergency Management*, Volume 8, Issue 1, Article 13, 2011.

Hoffman, D. E., "The Little Nukes That Got Away," *Foreign Policy.com*, April 2010.

Hospital Safety Center, HCPro, "Annual security assessments become California law," June 2010.

Hsu, S., "Pre-Katrina Emergency Plan for Elderly Faulted," *washingtonpost.com*, January 31, 2006.

Huser, T. J., "Suspect SARS patient puts hospital's plan on defense," *Journal of Healthcare Protection Management*, Volume 21, Number 1, Winter 2005.

Jarvis, R., "Katrina negligence lawsuit has implications for all hospitals" *usatoday.com*, January 11, 2010.

Johnson, K., "Staff at New Orleans hospital debated euthanizing patients," *CNN.com*, October 13, 2005

Johnson, K., Frank T., "Mumbai attacks refocus U.S. Cities," *usatoday.com*, December 5, 2008.

Joint Commission Online, "Accreditation: Measures of Success requirements deleted," *JointCommission.org*, April 2010.

Joint Commission, "Hospitals of the Future Report," *JointCommission.org*, November 2008.

Kauffman, T., "Plutonium spill, laser accident prompt reviews," *FederalTimes.com*, September 7, 2008.

Kavilanz, P., "U.S. To hospitals: Clean up your act," *CNN Money.com*, April 2010.

Kiltz, L., "Developing Critical Thinking Skills in Homeland Security and Emergency Management Courses," *Journal of Homeland Security and Emergency Management*, Volume 6, Issue 1, 2009.

Kimery, A., "DEMOCRATS, BI-PARTISAN REPORT SLAM ADMIN ON HOMELAND, NATIONAL SECURITY," *hstoday.us*, September 09, 2008.

Kliff, S., Skipp, C., "Overlooked: The Littlest Evacuees," *Newsweek*, October 6, 2008.

Kochems, A., "Who's on First/ A Strategy for Protecting Critical Infrastructure," *Backgrounder*, The Heritage Foundation, May, 2005.

Lurie, N., Wasserman, J., Nelson, C. D., "Preparedness: Evolution or Revolution?" *Health Affairs*, July/August 2005, Volume 25, Number 4.

Matessina, J., "From advocacy to emergency," *Modern Healthcare*, Opinion/Commentary, September 19, 2005.

McCarter M., "Dirty Bomb Recovery Plan Lacking," *hstoday.us*, March 1, 2010.

McCarter, M., "Officials Outline Terrorist Threats to United States," *hstoday.us*, October 2, 2009.

McFee, Dr. Robin, "On Terrorism: WMD Preparedness," IAHSS Directions, Volume 22, Number 1, *Journal of Healthcare Protection Management*, 2009.

McKinley, J. Jr., "Hospital flooded in storm to Cut Its Staff by a Third," *nytimes.com*, November 14, 2008.

McKinney, M., "Prepping for crisis-Study pokes holes in effort to combat threats," Sebelius, *Modern Healthcare*, Policy, October 4, 2010.

REFERENCES

McLaughlin, S., Spaanbroek, S., "We'll figure out what to do when the time comes: the need for developing effective emergency operation exercises," *Journal of Healthcare Protection Management*, Volume 25, Number 1, 2009.

Mculley, R., "Is New Orleans Having a Mental Breakdown?" *time.com*, Agust 01, 2006.

Michelman, B. S., "The Amazing Evolution of an Industry: Past, Present and Future of Healthcare Security," *Journal of Healthcare Protection Management*, Volume 20, Number 1, Winter 2002.

Moore, M., "Vigilance Reduces Vulnerabilities — Protect Your Hospital," *MATRIX*, Volume 2, Issue 2.

Morrow, A., "Deaths of Patients in Hurricane Katrina Aftermath: Disaster Casualties, Mercy Killing or Murder?," *dying.about.com*, September 16, 2006.

NBC News, "FBI: U.K. terror suspects tried to work in U.S.," July 2007.

NNSA Press Release, "NNSA works with New York City to Counter Radiological Threats," *nnsa.energy.gov*, July 06, 2010.

Ornstein, C., Webber, T., "Many California Health Workers Not Checked For Criminal Pasts," *L.A. Times*, December 2008.

Paddoc,M., "Funding & Resources: Emergency Healthcare's Unique Funding Track" *hstoday.us*, March 01, 2011.

Perry, R. W., Lindell, M. K., "Hospital Planning for Weapons of Mass Destruction," *Journal of Healthcare Protection Management*, Volume 23, Number 1, 2007.

Perry, T., Wilkinson, T., "Quake rolls across Baja," *latimes.com*, April, 2010.

Pettit, W. R., "Prepare Now for Pandemic Readiness Security and Patient Surge," *Journal of Healthcare Protection Management*, Volume 25, Number 2, 2009.

Phares, W., "Warning: The Jihadist are Mushrooming Inside America," *FamilySecurityMatters.org*, September 2009.

Ramirez, M., "The Unprepared Beware," *EzineArticles.com*, March 2007.

RAND CONGRESSIONAL RESOURCES, "Nearly Half of California Hospitals Unprepared to Meet Deadlines for Seismic Safety," *rand.org*, March, 2007.

Rauber, C., "Cal Pacific, Stanford hope to postpone huge seismic upgrades" *bizjournals.com*, August 20, 2010.

Reddy, S., "Hospitals likely to face litigation," *dallasnews.com*, September 15, 2005.

Reddy, S., "In Flood, hospital becomes a hell," *dallasnews.com*, September 4, 2005.

Rivers, S., Speraw, S., Phillips, K., Lee, J., "A Review of Nurses in Disaster Paredness and Response: Military and Civilian Collaboration" Volume 7, Issue 1, Article 61, *Journal of Homeland Security and Emergency Management*, 2010.

Robinson, L. A., Hammitt, J. K., Aldy, J. E., Krupnick, A., Baxter, J., "Valuing the Risk of Death from Terrorist Attacks," *Journal of Homeland Security and Emergency Management*, Volume 7, Issue 1, Article 14, 2010.

Rubin, J., "The proposed NIMS training Plan: What's going on?" *homeland1.com*, March 01, 2011.

REFERENCES

Ruquet, M., "$165 Billion Quake Looms For Bay Area," *propertyandcasualtyinsurancenews.com*, March 20, 2008.

Shadden, M., "Planning to Survive and Operate: Business Continuity," *Inside Homeland Security*, Volume 7, Issue 1, Spring 2009.

Smyth, J., "Violent assaults on ER nurses rise as programs cut," *msnbc.msm.com*, August 10, 2010.

Spencer, P., "The Security Case for Patient and Family Centered Care," *Journal of Healthcare Protection Management*, Volume 24, Number 2, 2008.

Stewart, S., "Dirty Bombs Revisited: Combating the Hype," *STRATFOR.com*, April 22, 2010.

Strohm, C., "Weather Services Officials gave dire, accurate warnings before Katrina hit," September 22, 2005.

TFAH, "On the Third Anniversary of Hurricane Katrina: Trust for America's Health Questions State of National Emergency preparedness," August 28, 2008.

The Associated Press, "19 Health Care Facilities Probed in La., *washingtompost.com*, October 3, 2005.

Thomas G., "MI5 Discover Al-Qaeda Buying Ambulances on Ebay" *G2 Magazine*, November 2008.

Trull, F., "Animal Rights Terrorism, Activists Have Used Increasingly Dangerous Tactics on Researchers Whose Goal is to Save Lives," *L.A. Times*, August 2008.

Wallask, S., "Five Lessons U.S. Hospitals Can Take from Haiti," *Health Leaders Media*, January 2010.

Weber, T., Ornstein, C., "State Fails to Report Disciplined Caregivers to Federal Database, *prorepublica.com*, July 19, 2010.

Webster, M., "Mexican Drug Cartel and Hezbollah Operating in Mexico and U.S.," *American Chronicle*, October 26, 2008.

Weinberger G., Joint Commission — April Changes to 2008 standards, April, 2008.

Wikipedia, "Hurricane preparedness for New Orleans" *Wikipedia.org*, September 1, 2005.

Williams, J. T., "Suicide bombers: Are you a target? What can you do?" *Journal of Healthcare Protection Management*, Volume 22, Number 2, 2006.

Yoker, B. C., Kizer, K. W., Lampe, P., Forrest, A. R. W., Lannan, J. M., Russell, D. A., "Serial Murder by Healthcare Professionals," *Journal of Healthcare Protection Management*, Volume 24, Number 1, 2008.

Zigmond, J., "Gulf Coast still hurting: Study," Modern Healthcare, *The Week in Healthcare*, August 28, 2006.

Zigmond, J., "Extreme Makeover, HHS should offer more emergency guidance: GAO," *ModernHealthcare.com*, February 1, 2010.

Zigmond, J., "Extreme makeover: HHS should offer more emergency guidance GAO, *modernhealthcare.com*, February 01, 2010.

Zigmond, J., "Life-altering decisions" *Modern Healthcare, Cover Story*, July 24, 2006.

Non-Author Reports

9/11 Commission Report, "Final report of the National Commission on Terrorist Attacks Upon the United States," 2004.

REFERENCES

Achenbach, J., "The Next Big One-where will it strike?," *National Geographic*, April 2006.

American Hospital Association, Final Report, Summary of an Invitational Forum, "Hospital Preparedness for Mass Casualties," August 2000.

Bradford D., Rubkin B., Viscardi P., White Paper Risk Management Series, "The New World of Extreme Risk: Terrorism Disaster Preparedness," *Advisen Ltd.*, October 2001.

Bradford, D., "Hospital Liability, Lessons Learned from Katrina, QuickNote, *Advisen Ltd.*, October 2005.

Defense Science Board, "Challenges to Military Operations in Support of U. S. Interests," Summer 2007 (Study Report).

DHHS Report, "The Next Challenge in Healthcare Preparedness: Catastrophic Health Events," Center for Biosecurity, UPMC, January 2010.

Fluman, A., Sanders, M., "Memorandum to Hospital Administrators, State and Local Emergency Managers and Public Health Directors," NIMS Compliance Activities. May 2006 (Memorandum).

Graham, B., Talent, J., "World at Risk: The Report of the Commission on the Prevention of Weapons of Mass Destruction Proliferation and Terrorism," December 2009.

Jewell, K., McGiffert L., "To Err is Human-To Delay is Deadly," Consumers Union, *SafePatientProject.org*, May 2009.

McCaffrey, B. R., "Strategic Challenges Facing the Obama Administration," PDF, *afa.org*, August 2009.

McFee, R., "Exclusive: Doctor Evil? Physicians & Scientists—Terrorists & Murderers in an Era of Global Terrorism" (part Three of Four).

Mead, C., Molander, R. C., "Considering the Effects of a Catastrophic Terrorist Attack," RAND Corporation, 2006.

President's Advisory Commission on Consumer Protection in the Health Care Industry, Final Meeting, March 1998.

Redlener, I., Johnson, D., Berman, D., Grant, R., "Follow-Up 2005: Where the American Public stands on Terrorism and Preparedness after Hurricane Katrina & Rita." *ncdp. mailman.columbia.edu*, 2005.

Rogers, M. C., "The Liability Risk of Hospitals as a Target of Terrorism," National Emergency Management Summit, Washington, D.C., February 2008 (Presentation).

Salinsky, E., "Strong as the Weakest Link: Medical Response to a Catastrophic Event," National Health Policy Forum, Background Paper—No. 65 August 8, 2008.

Southern Poverty Law Center, "Hate Group Numbers Up by 54% Since 2000," February 2009.

Suburban Emergency Management Project, "Lessons Learned from Hospital Evacuations during Tropical storm Allison," Biot Report #216: May 21, 2005.

Third Way, Center for American Progress Action Fund, "Homeland Security Presidential Transition Initiative," November 2008.

U.S. Department of Health and Human Services, "National Health Security Strategy of The United States of America," *hhs.org*. December 2009.

REFERENCES

U.S. Hearing: Subcommittee on Oversight and Investigations of the Committee on International Relations, "Visa Overstays: Can We Bar the Terrorist Door?" (109th Congress), May 2006.

U.S. House of Representatives Report 109-377, "A Failure of Initiative: Final Report of the Select Bipartisan Committee to Investigate the Preparedness for and Response to Hurricane Katrina," U.S. House of Representatives, 2006.

Union (AFL-CIO, AFSCME, AFT, CWA, SEUI, UAN, UFCW) Survey Report, "Healthcare Workers In Peril: Preparing To Protect Worker Health And Safety During Pandemic Influenza," April 2009.

AUTHOR PROFILE

James "Jim" Blair, DPA, MHA, FACHE, FABCHS, CMAS, is President of the Center for HeathCare Emergency Readiness (CHCER). He is a career-retired Army Colonel with 28 years of active service. He is a Korean War Era draftee trained as a combat Infantryman, combat medic and healthcare professional. His Army staff assignments include: Chief of Education and Training, Office of the Army Surgeon General; The Army Surgeon General's representative to the U.S. Army's reorganization of the Army Medical Department; Chief of Staff of 7th Medical Command and USAREUR Deputy Chief Surgeon for Medical Support Services. He served in the role of Chief Executive Officer in hospitals ranging from Combat Field and Combat Evacuation, Community, Medical Center and a Hospital System with two Medical Centers and Eleven Community Hospitals. He holds a number of combat awards.

Among his private sector experiences are Vice President, Hospital Corporation of America (HCA), Middle East Limited, Independent consultant to the Joint Commission International, Independent healthcare consulting to the Middle East and Africa, and Independent consultant to Native American Tribes under the Indian Sovereignty Act.

His Public Sector experiences include Deputy Director, South Carolina Health and Human Services Finance Commission. He holds a number of University Academic appointments. Dr. Blair is a member of Epsilon Phi Delta National Honor Society in Heath Administration and is the author of a recent Book on All-Hazards Healthcare Emergency Readiness. He is the author of numerous articles spanning a number of expert healthcare domains.